SURGERY - PROCEDURES, COMPLICATIONS, AND RESULTS

COMPUTER-ASSISTED SURGERY

NEW DEVELOPMENTS, APPLICATIONS AND POTENTIAL HAZARDS

Surgery - Procedures, Complications, and Results

Additional books in this series can be found on Nova's website under the Series tab.

Additional e-books in this series can be found on Nova's website under the e-book tab.

SURGERY - PROCEDURES, COMPLICATIONS, AND RESULTS

COMPUTER-ASSISTED SURGERY

NEW DEVELOPMENTS, APPLICATIONS AND POTENTIAL HAZARDS

XIAOJUN CHEN
EDITOR

NOVA BIOMEDICAL
New York

NOTICE TO THE READER

Library of Congress Cataloging-in-Publication Data

ISBN: 978-1-63463-811-1

Library of Congress Control Number: 2014958717

Published by Nova Science Publishers, Inc. † New York

CONTENTS

PREFACE

Nowadays, the computer-assisted surgery and the robot-assisted surgery are broadly used in the operating room to assist surgeons in improving accuracy and precision of procedures, producing more reliable and reproducible outcomes, minimizing the invasiveness of surgical procedures, and improving patient safety. In this book, the authors present current developments, applications and potential hazards in the domain of computer-aided surgery and robotic surgery. Topics in this compilation include surgical navigation system based on 3D Slicer using augmented reality (AR) technology; computer-assisted minimally invasive surgery; a navigation system in bimaxillary orthognathic surgery; spinal surgical navigation system; scrub nurse robot systems for laparoscopic surgery; ultrasound imaging for robotic orthopedic surgery, etc.

Chapter 1 introduces a surgical navigation module based on 3D Slicer using augmented reality (AR) technology. With the use of this system, including the calibration of instruments, registration, and the calibration of HMD, the 3D virtual critical anatomical structures are aligned with the actual structures of patient in real-world scenario during the intra-operative motion tracking process. Therefore, some disadvantages of the traditional surgical navigation (for example, the surgeon is no longer obliged to switch between the real operation scenario and computer screen) are overcome, and the safety, accuracy, and reliability of the surgery may be improved. Furthermore, this module could be shared with the global research community and extended to various surgeries.

Chapter 2 includes accessing the feasibility of the technique and evaluating the success rate of three different registration methods – facial surface registration, anatomic landmark-based registration, and template-based registration. Eighteen cases of facial surface-based registration, 63 cases of anatomic landmark-based registration, and 8 cases of template-based registration were analyzed. The overall success rate of facial surface-based registration was 39%, which was significant lower than template-based (100%, $p = 0.013$) and anatomic landmark-based registration (95%, $p < 0.0001$). And, the accuracy of image-guided maxillary positioning in the sagittal and vertical directions was evaluated. Student's two-tailed paired t-test was used to evaluate differences between the planned and actual surgical movement of the maxilla, which were 0.63 ± 0.50 mm (p = 0.12) in the sagittal direction and 0.57 ± 0.37 mm (p = 0.45) in the vertical direction. The results show that the navigation system is a useful perioperative tool to control the surgical change of the maxilla in bimaxillary surgery.

Chapter 3 focuses on the introduction of computer-assisted surgery, including image-guided surgery and robot-assisted surgery, to support surgical interventions has provided surgeons with new assistance tools to address the limitations of minimally invasive surgery (MIS) as well as improve the clinical results. These systems improve the surgeon perception of the patient anatomy and provide tools to analyze in advance the most suited approach to carry out the surgical intervention. And, augmented reality (AR) offers a suitable way to enhance the common view of the surgical field with useful information as preoperative images and virtual models. Although this technology is well established for rigid anatomy, further work has to be done for full integration with deformable anatomical models. Continuous technological advances in robotic-assisted surgery have led to potential improvements in the development of MIS procedures such as 3D vision, increased precision and dexterity, and ergonomic conditions for the surgeon.

Chapter 4 shares detailed methods about setting up a navigation system and the know how of using navigation systems, especially in minimally invasive spinal surgeries. The research team has already introduced skin fixed dynamic reference frame (DRF) into mini open transforaminal lumbar interbody fusion (TLIF) and recently examine accuracy of skin fixed DRF in anterior cervical foraminotomy. Both methods require only a few minutes to set up and do not prohibit the natural movement of the surgeon during the operation. With development of the navigation system, spine surgeon can perform complex and minimal invasive surgery successfully without radiation hazard.

Chapter 5 reviews the current approaches in robotic surgery, where ultrasound based navigation is used, with a special care on orthopedics. The control of robots is evolving at an enormous pace and is strongly pushed by the recent advances in medical imaging. Ultrasound imaging plays a decisive role in robotic surgery because it is less invasive and widely used by medical doctors. The main drawback is the precision of the measurements taken from US images. It is shown that this error is less than 2 mm nowadays, which allows it use in the operating room during surgeries. However, recent navigation systems are still slow, and cannot be operated in real-time, although they can give a measure to correct the robot trajectory. Future developments in this field will surely take care of diminishing the computational time, and also the precision of the system.

Chapter 6 shows the development of scrub nurse robot (SNR) systems for laparoscopic surgery. The SNR was designed to adapt to surgeons with various levels of skill and different personalities, and had a novel function: automatic insertion of a surgical instrument to achieve a smooth instrument exchange with the expectation that the higher functional ability would increase surgical operation efficacy. Three versions of SNR systems have already been developed for endoscopic and laparoscopic surgery so that the surgeons performing endoscopic and laparoscopic surgery do not use as many types of surgical instruments as in conventional surgery in which the abdominal or thoracic wall is cut open widely. Moreover, the goals of the SNR are for it to be able to accurately anticipate which instrument the surgeon will request for the next step of surgery and to hand this to the surgeon in a timely fashion.

Chapter 7 proposes a complete pipeline for image and shape analysis for the fluorescent T-cell images. In particular, researchers have used the Wasserstein 2-metric to measure the shape variation of the T-cells, which shows an interesting correlation with the intracellular calcium concentration. It is also noted that since both the Ca^2+ concentration and the shape metric computation depends upon the segmentation of the T-cells, the author's must consider the question of whether the correlation between the two measures is caused by the common segmentation upon which they are based.

In conclusion, computer-aided surgery and robotic surgery have experienced tremendous progress over the past decades by minimizing the risks and improving the precision of the surgery. However, the development of this kind of technology is still under way. In the future, the performance of the computer-aided system will be greatly enhanced, for example, higher precision, more intelligent automation, more friendly user interface, etc., and it will become increasingly popular in hospitals.

In: Computer-Assisted Surgery
Editor: Xiaojun Chen
ISBN: 978-1-63463-811-1

Chapter 1

DEVELOPMENT OF A SURGICAL NAVIGATION SYSTEM BASED ON 3D SLICER USING AUGMENTED REALITY (AR) TECHNOLOGY

Xiaojun Chen * ***and Lu Xu***
Institute of Biomedical Manufacturing and Life Quality Engineering, School of Mechanical Engineering, Shanghai Jiao Tong University, Shanghai, China

ABSTRACT

Over the past decades, the field of computer-aided surgery has experienced tremendous development due to the rapid growth of computing power and the improvements in imaging modalities [1]. Based on the guidance of preoperative planning with CT, magnetic resonance imaging (MRI), or other volumetric image data associated with the patient, surgical navigation system is being widely used in various surgeries (ear, nose, oral implantology, etc.) for minimizing the risks and improving the precision of the surgeries [2]. Although some commercially-available surgical navigation systems have been approved for clinical applications, these systems are expensive and not open to the public. 3D Slicer is a free open source software platform for the research

* Correspondence to: Xiaojun Chen, PhD; Room 805, School of Mechanical Engineering, Shanghai Jiao Tong University, Dongchuan Road 800, Minhang District, Shanghai, China; Post Code: 200240; E-mail: xiaojunchen@163.com; Tel: (+86) -13472889728, (+86) 21-62816517; Fax: (+86)21-34206847.

community of computer-aided surgery. In this contribution, a loadable module based on Slicer to support surgical navigation has been developed and validated. This research module allows reliable calibration of the surgical instruments, point-based registration and surface matching registration, so that the position and orientation of the surgical instrument can be tracked and displayed on the computer screen in real time to reduce the surgical risks. Furthermore, this module could be shared with global research community and be extended to various surgeries. On the other hand, Augmented Reality (AR)-based surgical navigation is a promising technology for clinical applications. For example, virtual anatomical structures such as soft tissues, blood vessels and nerves can be integrated with the real-world scenario in real time. In this study, an AR-based surgical navigation module (AR-SNS) is developed using an optical see-through HMD (head-mounted display), aiming at improving the safety and reliability of the surgery. With the use of this system, including the calibration of instruments, registration, and the calibration of HMD, the 3D virtual critical anatomical structures are aligned with the actual structures of patient in real-world scenario during the intra-operative motion tracking process.

Keywords: Computer-aided surgery, 3D slicer, augmented reality, optical see-through HMD

1. INTRODUCTION

Percutaneous sacroiliac joint screw fixation is a kind of minimally invasive surgery for the clinical treatment of posterior pelvic ring injury. Compared with the traditional open reduction and internal fixation, the advantage of the screw insertion technique is that it brings less trauma, less intra-operative blood loss, low infection rate and necrosis rate, quick recovery, etc. However, in order to avoid injuring the peripheral nerves, blood vessels and soft tissues, it is important to control the position and orientation of screw through the intra-operative guidance. Currently, the major techniques include the X-ray C-arm system and computer-aided surgical navigation. Compared with the traditional X-ray C-arm system, the 2D or 3D computer-aided navigation system can improve the safety of sacroiliac joint screw insertion significantly and reduce the intra-operative X-ray fluoroscopy time.

Over the past decades, the field of computer-aided surgery has experienced tremendous development due to the rapid growth of computing power and the improvements in imaging modalities [1]. Based on the guidance of preoperative planning with CT, magnetic resonance imaging (MRI), or other volumetric image data associated with the patient, surgical navigation system is being widely used in various surgeries (ear, nose, oral implantology, etc.) for minimizing the risks and improving the precision of the surgeries [2]. Although some commercially-available surgical navigation systems have been approved for clinical applications such as Kick (Brainlab, Germany), StealthStation (Medtronic, USA), eNLight and NavSuite (Stryker Corporation, USA), Navigation Panel Unit (Storz, Germany) and etc., [3], the disadvantages include high-cost of the whole system and failure to clarify the several apparent issues pertaining to the calibration of the surgical instrument, registration, intra-operative motion tracking, etc. [2] In 2012, Daniel Behrendt (University of Leipzig, Germany), Martin Koestler (BrainLAB, Germany), et al. [4] evaluated 2D-navigation and 3D-navigation for iliosacral screw fixation using the commercial computer-aided navigation systems (BrainLAB Trauma 2.6 and BrainLAB Spine & Trauma Fluoro-3D 1.6.0). However, the high cost of this navigation system restricts its wide clinical applications since it is not open to the public.

In this study, a powerful software package for visualization and medical image computing called Slicer, or 3D Slicer (Brigham Women's Hospital, Boston, MA) was used as a platform for developing a surgical navigation system. Unlike general commercial workstation, 3D Slicer is a free, open source software and is not required to specific hardware. The purpose of this study is to develop and evaluate a new loadable module named "Surgical Navigation System" (SNS) based on Slicer so that the risks of percutaneous implantation of sacroiliac joint screw surgery can be reduced in anatomically complex operation sites.

On the other hand, all of the traditional navigation systems use computer screen to render the navigation information such as the real-time position and orientation of the surgical instrument, virtual path of preoperative surgical planning, and etc., so that the surgeons have to switch between the actual operation site and computer screen which is inconvenient and impact the continuity of surgery.

In recent years, due to the great development of Augmented Reality (AR) technology, more and more wearable AR devices have appeared like Google Glass, Skully AR-1 (An AR motorcycle helmet) [5], and etc. AR is an integrated technique of image processing, and in AR system, real objects and virtual (computer-generated) objects are combined in a real environment. Furthermore, real and virtual objects are aligned with each other, and run interactively in real time [6, 7]. Due to the advantages of AR visualization, developing a surgical navigation system based on AR is a significant challenge for the next generation. For example, after the registration of the preoperative CT in relation to the intra-operative realistic scene, surgeons can superimpose the virtual CT data onto the patient's anatomy [8]. In 2010, Liao et al. [9, 10] developed a 3-D augmented reality navigation system for MRI-guided surgery by using auto-stereoscopic images, and the system creates a 3D image, fixed in space, which is independent of viewer pose. In addition, Navab et al. [11] from Technical University of Munich have demonstrated a very practical application of AR. They developed an X-ray C-arm system equipped with a video camera, so that a fused image that combines a direct video view of a patient's elbow with the registered X-ray image of the humerus, radius, and ulna bones was produced.

This study also presents an AR-based surgical navigation module (AR-SNS) using an optical see-through HMD (head-mounted display), which encompasses the preoperative surgical planning, registration, and intraoperative tracking. With the aid of AR-SNS, the surgeon wearing the HMD can obtain a fused image that virtual anatomical structures such as soft tissues, blood vessels and nerves integrated with the intra-operative real-world scenario, so that the safety and reliability of the surgery can be improved.

2. Methods and Materials

2.1. Surgical Navigation System Based on 3D Slicer

2.1.1. The Navigation Software Workflow Based on Slicer

Figure 1 shows the workflow and functions of the surgical navigation software based on Slicer (green) and the supporting algorithms and techniques (yellow). With the support of "SNS" module (pink) and some relevant modules from Slicer (blue), the 3D medical modeling, preoperative surgical planning, calibration of surgical instruments, registration, and intraoperative tracking can be realized. The framework of the software starts with loading of the preoperative CT data, and ends with the real-time navigation and its details described as follows:

1) Loading of the original CT data: The patient is imaged in the CT scanner, and the acquired images are automatically transferred to the Slicer interface via the "DICOM" module since Slicer allows loading

images in DICOM format from disk or directly from the clinical Picture Archiving and Communication System (PACS).

2) Image processing: Based on the CT data, each image can be segmented via the "Editor" module. Slicer provides different image segmentation methods for satisfying different requirements such as threshold segmentation and manual modification, so that the hard tissues and soft tissues can be marked.
3) 3D-Reconstruction: After image segmentation, a 3D surface model is reconstructed using the Marching Cubes algorithm [12]. All of the 3D modeling in this step is processed through the "Models" module of 3D Slicer.
4) Preoperative planning: Then, on the basis of these CT images and the 3D model, the user can implement preoperative surgical planning and 3D geometrical measurement via the Slicer ruler. When one target point and one entry point are selected, user can create a trajectory that connects these two points and adjust it in real-time. The virtual optimal path will be rendered on all of the 2D/3D views.
5) Communicate with optical tracking device: The Polaris Vicra optical tracking device can be activated and initialized via the "SNS" module.
6) Calibration of the surgical instruments: Since the Polaris optical tracking system only localizes the reference frame with mounted sphere-shaped retro-reflective markers, it is necessary to determine the spatial relationship between the surgical instrument and the reference frame (this procedure is also called as "calibration"). Figure 2 shows a simulated surgical drill and a simulated surgical saw used in this research and the coordinate systems for the instrument and the reference frame are respectively established. The calibration encompasses three sections, "Pivot Calibration", "Axis Calibration of surgical drill" and "Surface Calibration of surgical saw", so that the movements of the reference frame can represent those of the surgical instrument.
7) Registration: The basic requirement of any navigation technique is the registration, which is the process of bringing two coordinate systems into spatial alignment [1]. In the most common clinical scenario, patient's position must be registered (aligned) with preoperative image data set on the procedure table. There are a variety of registration methods including paired points [13-15] and surface matching [16, 17] concepts, which are proposed in this study. The details of registration are described below.

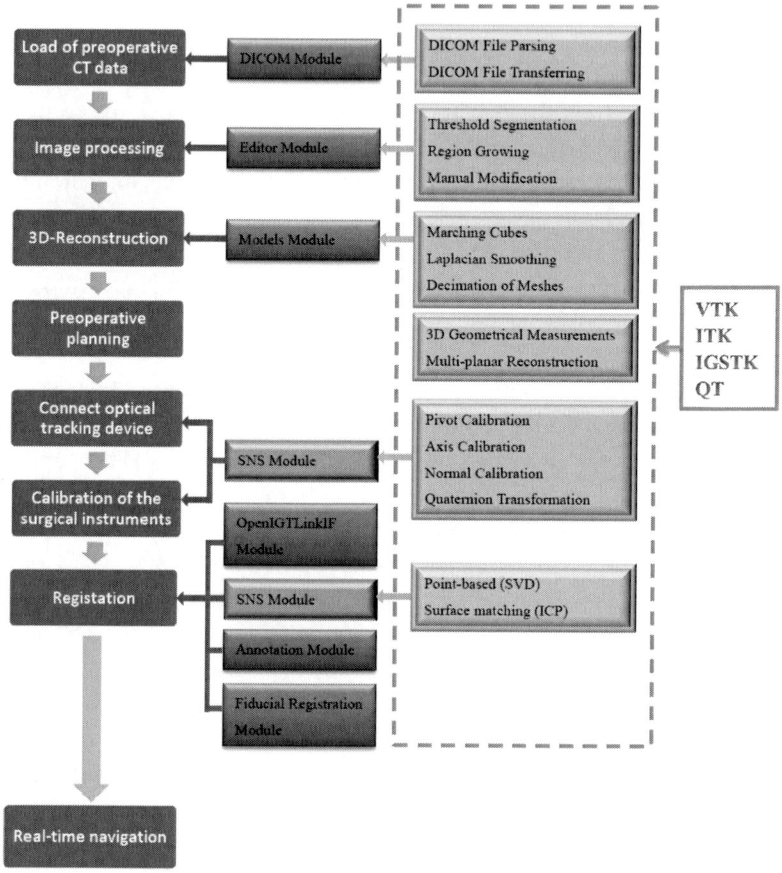

Figure 1. The workflow and functions of surgical navigation software based on Slicer.

2.1.2. Calibration of the Surgical Instruments

The "Pivot Calibration" is to calculate the offset values of the tip point of the instrument. This procedure can be realized through the following method. Pivot the surgical instrument slowly around the tip for about half a minute in the Polaris optical tracking system. Then, on the basis of the collected data of about 250 frames regarding to the movements of the reference frame, the offset values can be calculated. As for the detailed description of the involved algorithms during this procedure, please refer to Ref. [18]. An open-source C++ software library named Image-Guided Surgery Toolkit (IGSTK) providing classes for implementing the standard "Pivot Calibration" [19, 20] is applied to "SNS" module, and the calibration data is automatically saved into an XML file. The orientation of the surgical drill is very important to the surgeons. Figure 3 shows a calibration tool used in this study for carrying out the "Axis Calibration of surgical drill". There is a series of axial holes matched to the different drills. During the calibration process, the surgical drill is inserted into the matched axial hole, and the direction vector (u,v,w) of surgical drill relative to the coordinate system of reference frame can be obtained with the support of the tracking device (shown in Figure 4). According to (1), T1 and T2 are, respectively, the translation matrices of surgical drill's reference frame and calibration tool relative to the tracking system, and (1,0,0)T is the direction vector of axial hole in the coordinate system of calibration tool.

$$(u, v, w)^T = T_I^{-1} T_2 \begin{bmatrix} 1 \\ 0 \\ 0 \end{bmatrix} \quad (1)$$

As for the "Surface Calibration of surgical saw", Figure 5 shows the calibration. The handpiece of the saw lies on the two v grooves, and the blade is inserted into the slot of the calibration tool. The axial vector of the v groove and normal vector of the slot under the coordinate system of calibration tool are all known, and with the support of the tracking device, the normal vector $(u_x, v_x, w_x)^T$ and axial vector $(u_y, v_y, w_y)^T$ of surgical saw relative to the reference frame can be calculated as follows:

$$(u_x, v_x, w_x)^T = T_I^{-1} T_2 \begin{bmatrix} 1 \\ 0 \\ 0 \end{bmatrix} \quad (2)$$

$$(u_y, v_y, w_y)^T = T_I^{-1} T_2 \begin{bmatrix} 0 \\ 1 \\ 0 \end{bmatrix} \quad (3)$$

According to (2) and (3), T_I and T_2 are, respectively, the translation matrices of surgical saw's reference frame and calibration tool relative to the tracking system. $(1,0,0)^T$ and $(0,1,0)^T$ are, respectively, the normal vector of slot and axial vector of v groove in the coordinate system of calibration tool.

Since the quaternion is used in the XML file to presents the axial offset values while the initial calibrated results are vectors, we need to transform the vectors to a quaternion before running the tracking system. Based on the extension of Euler's formula, a quaternion (shown in (5)) can represents any rotation in three dimensions with an angle of rotation of θ around the axis defined by a unit vector see (4).

$$\underset{u}{\rightarrow} = (u_x, u_y, u_z) = u_x\mathrm{i} + u_y\mathrm{j} + u_z\mathrm{k} \tag{4}$$

$$\mathrm{q} = \cos\frac{1}{2}\theta + (u_x\mathrm{i} + u_y\mathrm{j} + u_z\mathrm{k})\sin\frac{1}{2}\theta \tag{5}$$

Suppose $\underset{v}{\rightarrow}$ is the obtained vector value when calibration step is completed:

$$\underset{v}{\rightarrow} = (\underset{v_x}{\rightarrow}\underset{v_y}{\rightarrow}\underset{v_z}{\rightarrow}) \tag{6}$$

And in this study, a 3D simulated instrument model is built along the negative direction of Z axis; thus:

$$\underset{z}{\rightarrow} = \left(\underset{z_x}{\rightarrow}\underset{z_y}{\rightarrow}\underset{z_z}{\rightarrow}\right) = (0, 0, -1) \tag{7}$$

Since the unit vector $\underset{u}{\rightarrow}$ equals the cross product of vector $\underset{v}{\rightarrow}$ and $\underset{z}{\rightarrow}$, based on the (8):

$$\begin{aligned} \underset{u}{\rightarrow} = \underset{z}{\rightarrow} \times \underset{v}{\rightarrow} &= \begin{vmatrix} \mathrm{i} & \mathrm{j} & \mathrm{k} \\ z_x & z_y & z_z \\ v_x & v_y & v_z \end{vmatrix} \\ &= \begin{vmatrix} z_y & z_z \\ v_y & v_z \end{vmatrix}\mathrm{i} - \begin{vmatrix} z_x & z_z \\ v_x & v_z \end{vmatrix}\mathrm{j} + \begin{vmatrix} z_x & z_y \\ v_x & v_y \end{vmatrix}\mathrm{k} \end{aligned} \tag{8}$$

Hence:

$$\cos\theta = \frac{\underset{z}{\rightarrow}\cdot\underset{v}{\rightarrow}}{\|\underset{z}{\rightarrow}\|\,\|\underset{v}{\rightarrow}\|} = \frac{\underset{z_x}{\rightarrow}\underset{v_x}{\rightarrow} + \underset{z_y}{\rightarrow}\underset{v_y}{\rightarrow} + \underset{z_z}{\rightarrow}\underset{v_z}{\rightarrow}}{\sqrt{z_x^2+z_y^2+z_z^2} \times \sqrt{v_x^2+v_y^2+v_z^2}} \tag{9}$$

So according to (8) and (9), $\underset{u}{\rightarrow}$, $\cos\frac{1}{2}\theta$, $\sin\frac{1}{2}\theta$ are all known , substitution of these results into (5) leads to the value of q. And the quaternion q can be finally written into the XLM file and be read when the Polaris optical tracking system is running.

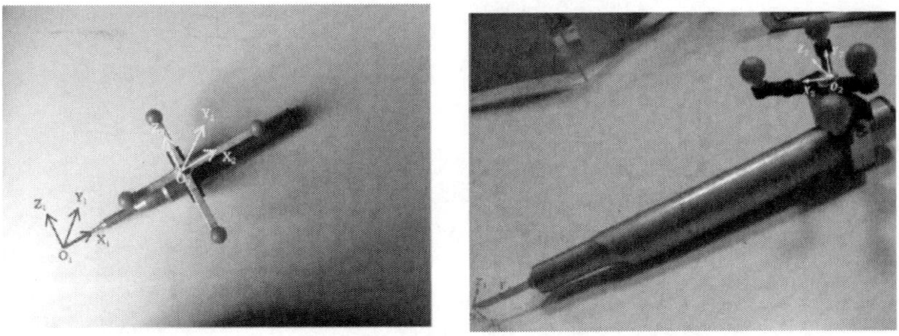

a) the coordinate systems of surgical drill and the reference

b) the coordinate systems of surgical saw and the reference

Figure 2. The simulated surgical instruments used in this research.

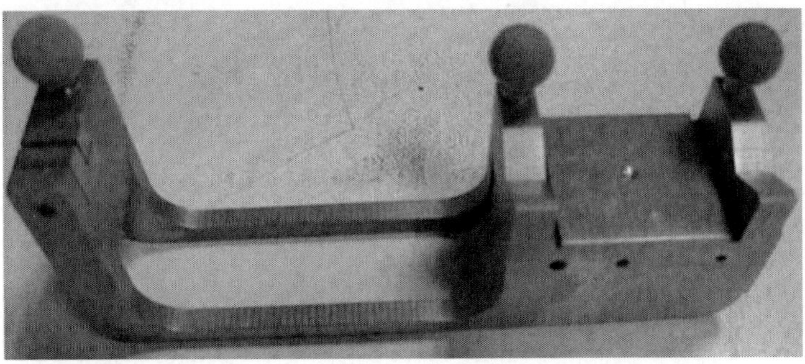

Figure 3. The calibration tool.

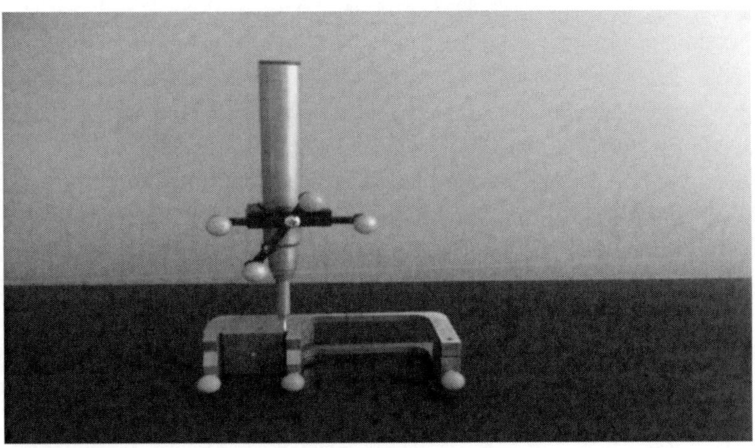

Figure 4. The calibration for the surgical drill axis.

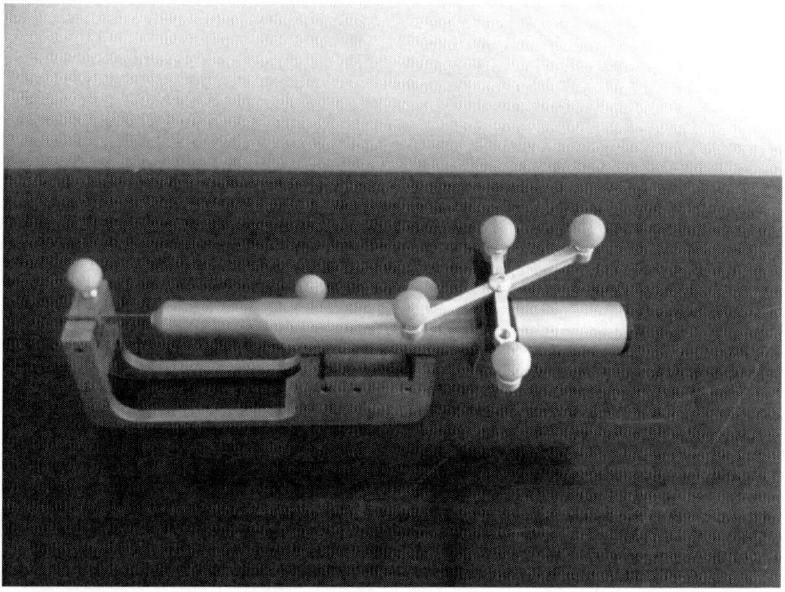

Figure 5. The calibration for the surgical saw surface.

2.1.3. Registration

Figure 6 shows the establishment of coordinate systems for real-time tracking in Slicer. There are four 3D coordinate systems, respectively, world coordinate system XYZ determined by the optical tracing system; virtual coordinate system $X_0Y_0Z_0$ (also referred as to the image coordinate system) determined by Slicer; reference coordinate system 1 $X_1Y_1Z_1$ (also referred as to the patient coordinate system) determined by the reference frame fixed on the patient; reference coordinate system 2 $X_2Y_2Z_2$ determined by the position probe. A1 and A2 are the transformation matrices with which Reference Coordinate System 1-2 can be, respectively, transformed to world coordinate system, and are all known through the Polaris optical tracking system. A0 and A10 are the registration transformation matrices with which world coordinate system and reference coordinate system 1 can be, respectively, transformed to virtual coordinate system, and can be obtained through singular value decomposition (SVD) algorithm. Therefore, the spatial relationship among the various coordinate systems in navigation system can be determined, so that the movements of the patient and surgical instruments can be rendered in the preoperative image coordinate system in real time. As for the detailed principle of the point-based registration, please refer to [21].

In Slicer, the point-based registration step is accomplished using the "OpenIGTLinkIF", "SNS", "Annotation" and "Fiducial Registration" modules in 3D Slicer. The "OpenIGTLinkIF" module is a program module for network communication with external software/hardware using OpenIGTLink protocol. Therefore, with the support of this module, the optical tracking device can be connected, and it can implement the import and export of position, linear transform and image data between OpenIGTLinkIF-compliant software and MRML scene [22]. MRML scene is a coherent internal data structure that maintains the links between the individual medical image data types, their visualization and any other steady state of the application and modules. While the tracking device Polaris Vicra is communicated with Slicer through the "OpenIGTLinkIF", the "SNS" will help the user to obtain a list of fiducial coordinates in the realistic world that matched with the fiducials picked on the virtual image. Based on the two matched lists of fiducials in "Annotation", the fiducial registration can be completed and the position and orientation of the surgical instrument model varies on the computer screen in real time so that the navigation procedure is realized.

Paul J. Besl and Neil D. Mckay [23] described a general-purpose, representation-independent method based on the iterative closest point (ICP) algorithm for registration of 3-D shapes, which is widely used in the field of medical image registration. Therefore, in order to improve the registration precision, surface-based registration based on ICP is realized in "SNS" module. The principle of this method is seeking the closest measured point corresponding with target point set though the repeated iteration. It is an optimal matching algorithm based on the least square method, and the registration is accomplished while the value of objective function that residual sum of squares formed is less than the preset threshold. Figure 7 shows the point cloud on the STL model for surface registration which is collected on the pelvic model surface of patient by using the positioning probe.

2.1.4. Phantom Experiment

In order to evaluate the feasibility of the navigation system, a rapid plastic pelvis model is used for conducting a phantom experiment. First, a 3D model was reconstructed through the "Models" module based on the CT data. Then, the calibration of instruments including the positioning probe and the surgical drill were completed in the "SNS" module. After the Polaris optical tracking device was communicated with Slicer through the "OpenIGTLinkIF" module, the operator created a list in "Annotation" module including three fiducials whose coordinates were all initially at origin of a virtual coordinate system

(VCS). Meanwhile, with the application of the Polaris and the positioning probe (shown in Figure 8), the coordinates of the fiducials under the reference coordinate system (RCS) which was determined by the reference frame fixed on the pelvis model were also obtained. Using this two paired list of fiducial points (shown in Figure 9), a registration transformation matrix can be generated through the "Fiducial Registration" module and the movements of the surgical instruments now can be rendered in the preoperative image coordinate system in real time (see Figure 10). In addition, the "Volume Reslice Driver" module can reslice a volumetric image of the patient with the plane along the surgical tool and visualize the sectional image on the 2D and 3D viewer on the 3D Slicer window, which is particularly useful for stereotactic surgical navigation (also see Figure 10).

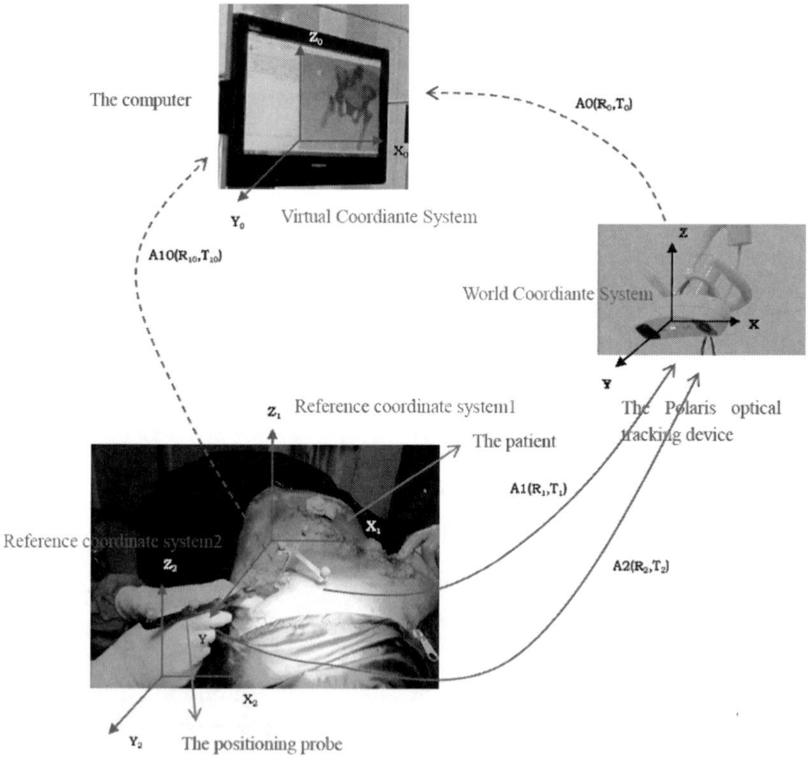

Figure 6. The establishment of coordinate systems for real-time tracking in Slicer.

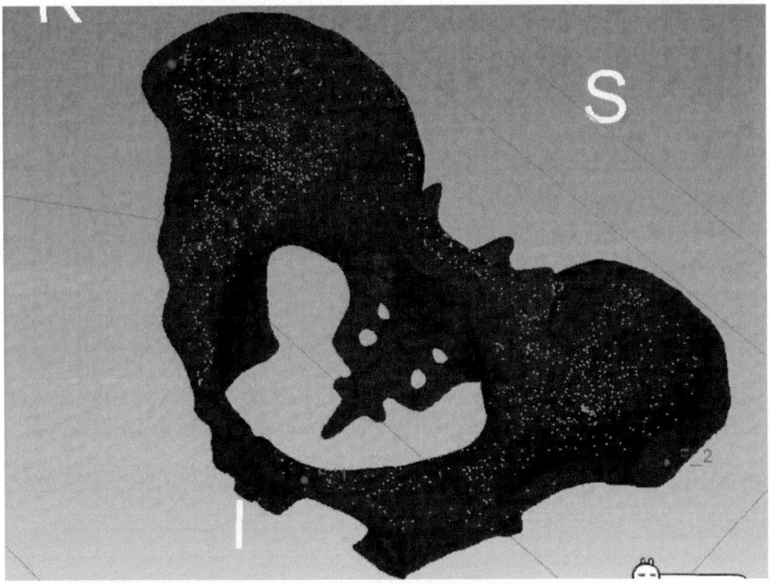

Figure 7. The point cloud for surface registration.

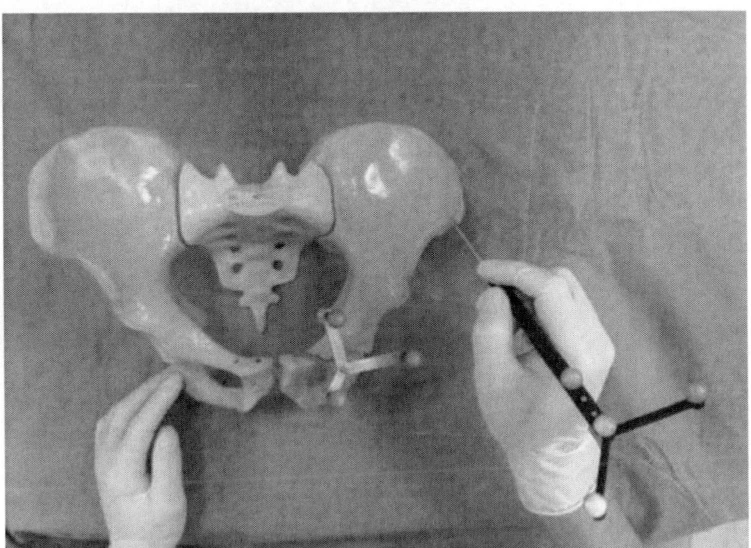

Figure 8. Using a positioning probe to collect the coordinates of the fiducial points.

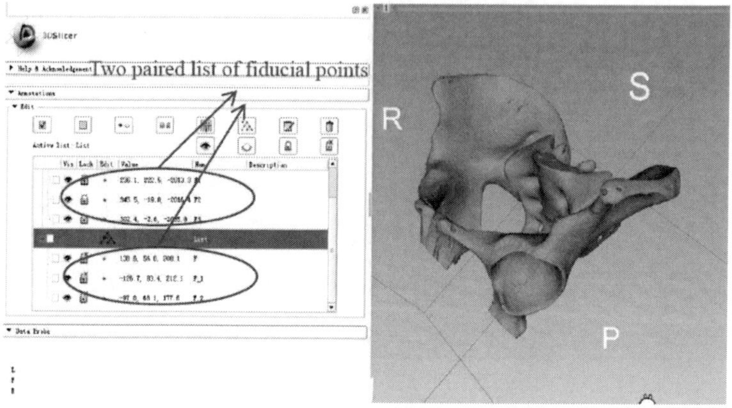

Figure 9. Two paired list of fiducial points.

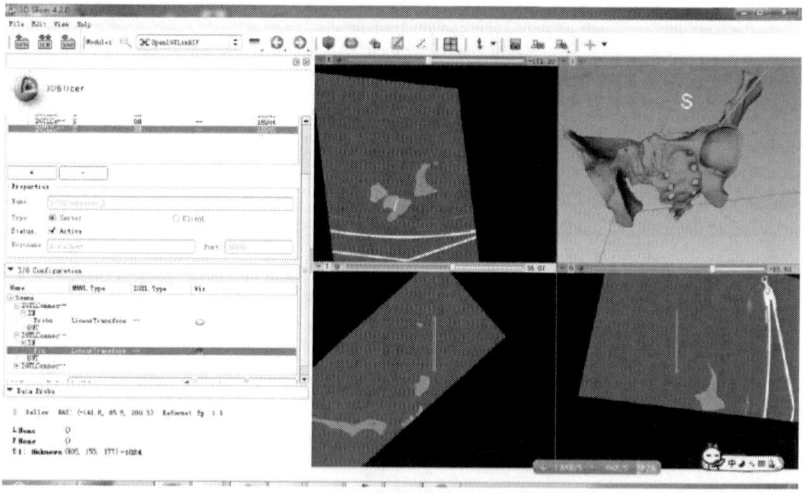

Figure 10. The position of the drill is tracked and rendered on the computer screen.

2.2. The AR-Based Surgical Navigation Module (AR-SNS)

2.2.1. The Hardware Architecture of AR-SNS

The AR-SNS is constructed based on a high-performance graphical workstation (HP), a 2D LCD monitor (G2200W, BenQ), an optical tracking device (Polaris Vicra, NDI Inc., Canada) and an optical see-through HMD (nVisor ST60, NVIS, United States) (Shown in Figure 11). The workstation is equipped with a 4GB memory card, a core i7 CPU and an nVIDIA Quadro FX4800 graphic card, running on the windows 7 operating system. As for HMD, it uses high-resolution microdisplays featuring 1280×1024 24-bit color pixels per eye, for vivid visual rendering and integration with reality.

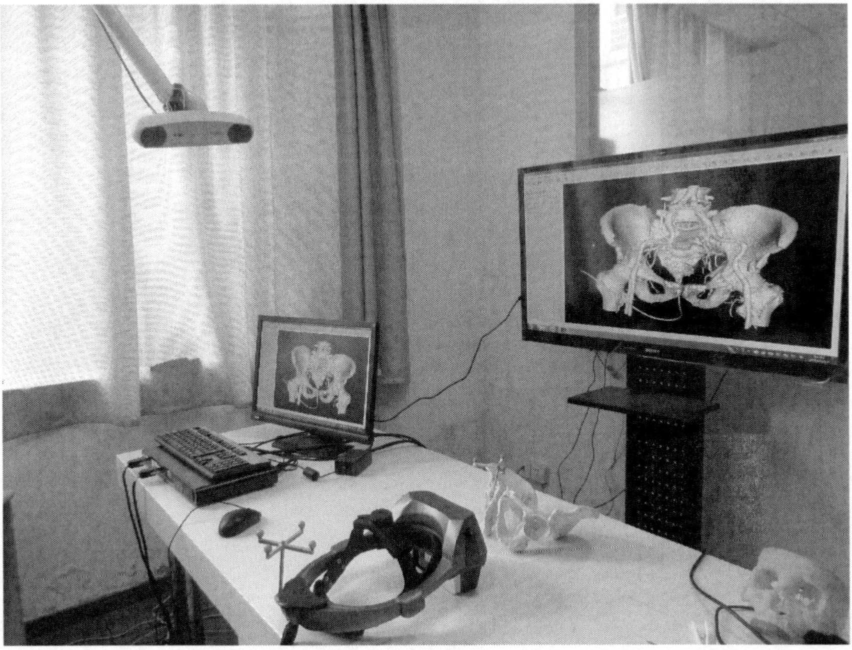

Figure 11. The hardware of AR-SNS.

2.2.2. 3d-Reconstruction and Preoperative Surgical Planning

Based on the original CT data, the segmentation of the hard tissue is conducted by using a threshold and region growing combined method, and for the soft tissue in each image, semi-automatic region growing method is adopted, and if it is over-segmented or under-segmented, manual modification is also used. Then, 3D surface models can be reconstructed through the marching cubes algorithm [12]. Figure 12 shows a 3D pelvis model and a bladder imported into AR-SNS after the 3D-reconstruction. All of the work including the image segmentation and 3D modeling is realized.

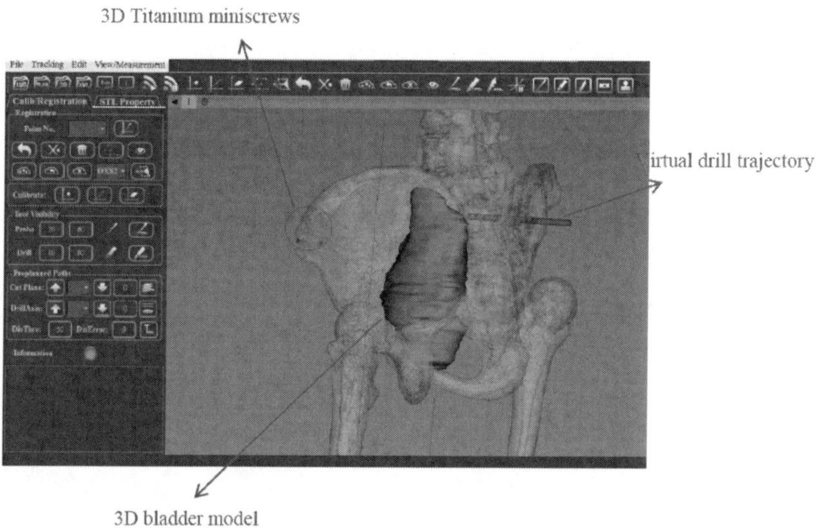

Figure 12. A 3D pelvis model and a bladder imported into the AR-SNS.

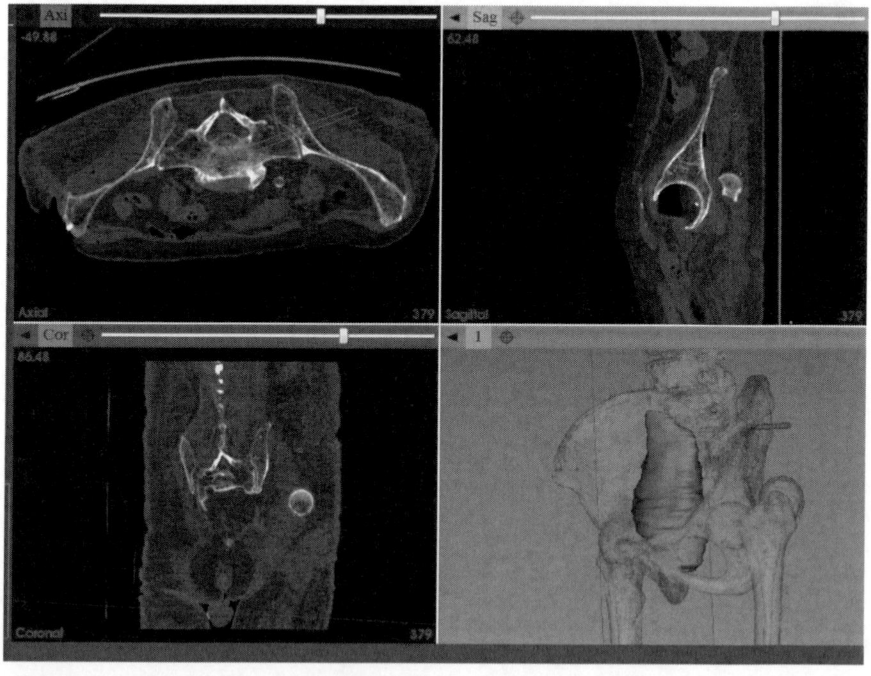

Figure 13. A virtual path for the surgical drill rendering on all of the 2D/3D views.

On the basis of these CT images and the 3D model, the procedure of preoperative planning can be implemented and is describe as follows: percutaneous implantation of sacroiliac joint screw is a very common surgery in orthopedics. And, in order to avoid injuring the important anatomical structures like soft tissues, blood vessels and nerves, a virtual path for the surgical drill should be created and will be rendered on all of the 2D/3D views. An example for a preoperative surgical planning is shown in Figure 13, so that the precision, safety and reliability of the implant surgery can be enhanced.

2.2.3. Calibration of the Patient's Position in Relation to the HMD

After registration, the preoperative images in HMD are aligned with the patient on the procedure table. Then, the calibration of HMD needs to be done. In the AR-SNS, the basic requirement is the calibration of the patient's position in relation to the HMD, which means the movement of the patient or the HMD will not affect the initial correspondence of VCS and RCS. The principle is described as follows: first of all, two reference frames are respectively mounted on the HMD and patient. Then, in order to obtain the calibration matrix after the initial registration of the patient's position in relation to the image data set, we built the transformation relationship shown in Figure 14. Suppose:

R is the initial transformation matrix of VCS to reference frame coordinate system2;

A_1 and A_2 are respectively the transformation matrix of reference frame coordinate system1 to the World Coordinate System before and after movement of the user head;

A_3 and A_4 are respectively the transformation matrix of reference frame coordinate system2 to the World Coordinate System before and after movement of the patient;

B_1 is the matrix of virtual model under the VCS before movement;

B_2 is the calibration transformation matrix of virtual model under the VCS.

Since the relative position of one point on the computer virtual image is fixed before and after movement, setting X as the coordinate of this point in computer virtual image coordinate system. Then, X_1 is the coordinate of X in VCS (also referred as the computer screen coordinate system) before movement and X_2 is the coordinate of X in VCS after movement. Equations (1) and (2) demonstrate the transformational relation:

$$RB_1X = X_1 \tag{1}$$

$$RB_2X = X_2 \tag{2}$$

The purpose is to maintain the relative position of this point in patient coordinate system unchanged before and after movement, so setting X3 as the coordinate of X in reference frame coordinate system2. Equations (3) and (4) show the transformational relation before and after movement:

$$(A_3)^{-1}A_1X_1 = X_3 \tag{3}$$

$$(A_4)^{-1}A_2X_2 = X_3 \tag{4}$$

Thus, based on Equations (1), (2), (3) and (4):

$$B_2 = [(A_4)^{-1}A_2R]^{-1}(A_3)^{-1}A_1RB_1 \tag{5}$$

In the polaris optical tracking system, seven elements representing the unit quaternion and the translation vector, are used to describe the transformation of a rigid body under world coordinate system. Therefore, A1, A2, A3, and A4 can be calculated on the basis of each rigid body's seven elements provided by the Polaris, and R can be calculated through the point-based registration and surface registration respectively under patient coordinate system and virtual coordinate system.

Since A_1, A_2, A_3, A_4, R, B_1 (which can be supposed as an identity matrix) are all known, the calibration transformation matrix B_2 can be calculated according to equation (5). As a result, the position and orientation of the virtual model will change with corresponds to the movement of HMD and patient, and match the real anatomical structures during intra-operative navigation procedure.

The setup of the AR-SNS and the actual view seen from the HMD is also illustrated in Figure 15.

2.2.4. Phantom Experiment and Cadaver Experiment

A phantom experiment was first conducted. With the original CT data (0.625 mm slice thickness, 512 × 512 matrix), a 3D pelvis model was reconstructed through the threshold segmentation, and fabricated using 3D printing technology. Then, the critical anatomical structures (especially the soft tissues, blood vessels and nerves) can be segmented using the manual modification method. In this experiment, a 3D bladder and some blood vessels and nerves were reconstructed. After calibration and registration, the AR-based surgical navigation was realized. Seen through the HMD, the 3D virtual anatomical structures were aligned with the real plastic pelvis model in any time regardless of the movement of HMD and model. (see Figure 15)

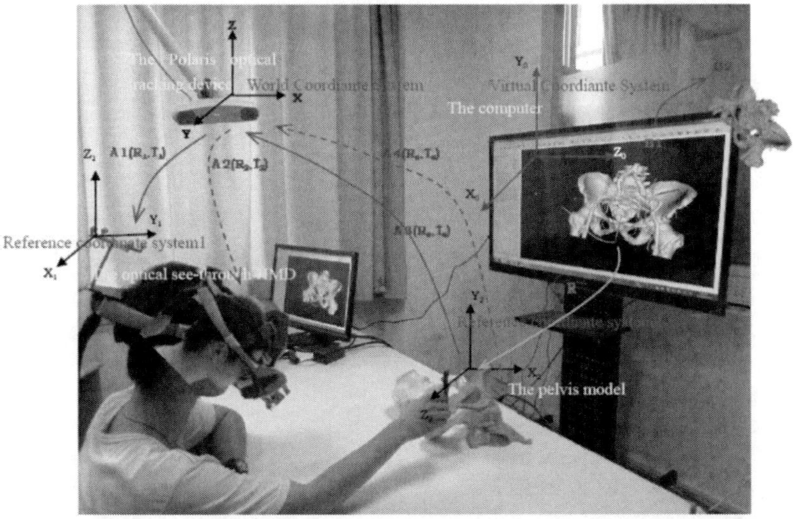

Figure 14. The establishment of coordinate systems in AR-SNS.

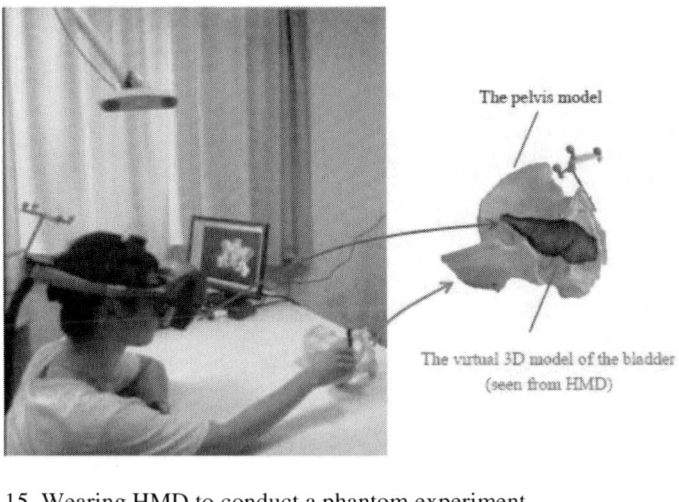

Figure 15. Wearing HMD to conduct a phantom experiment.

Researchers have also conducted a cadaver experiment for percutaneous implantation of sacroiliac joint screw in an operating room. First of all, five titanium miniscrews were inserted into the pelvis before CT scanning for fiducial point registration. Then, based on the CT data, 3D-reconstruction and preoperative surgical planning were conducted, and the data were imported to AR-SNS. Figure 12 shows the 3D-reconstruction, including a pelvis model, a bladder model and titanium miniscrews models. In addition, the optimization design of a virtual drill trajectory is the preoperative planning result. (see Figure 13) Then, in order to show the position and orientation of the surgical drill model correctly, point calibration and axis calibration were carried out. After point-based and surface matching registration and calibration of the HMD, the 3D virtual bladder was aligned with the real cadaveric pelvis during the intra-operative, and the 3D instrument model is displaying in HMD in real time, so that the operator can implant the sacroiliac joint screw into the pelvis along with the preoperative planned trajectory. (see Figure 16)

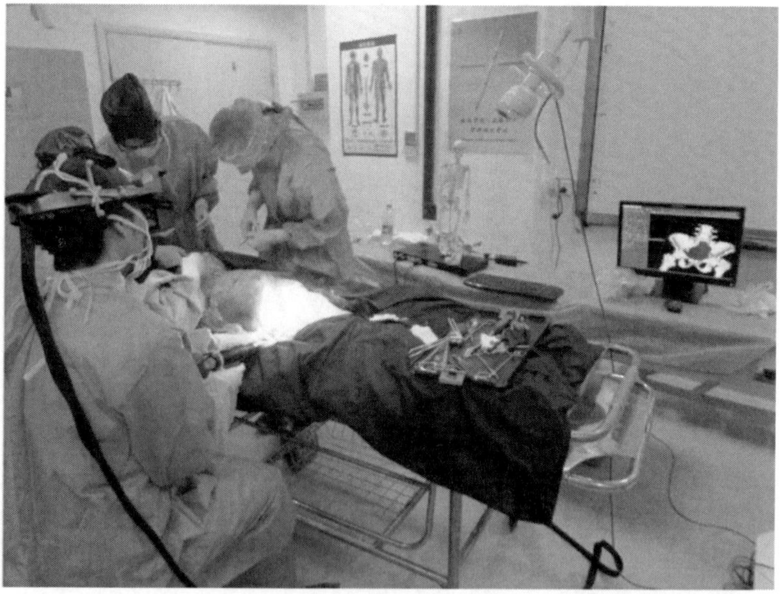

Figure 16. The panoramic view of the operating room for a cadaver experiment.

CONCLUSION

Nowadays, the minimally invasive surgery is becoming more and more popular in orthopaedics. Percutaneous implantation of sacroiliac joint screw is a typical surgery to treat the posterior pelvic ring injury. Nevertheless, due to the anatomic intricacies of the pelvis and the screw length, it is still a challenge to control the intra-operative position and orientation of the screw for avoiding damaging the surrounding critical anatomical structures. Furthermore, the radiation exposure of the conventional technique using intra-operative X-ray C-arm system is excessive. In the past years, an image-guided system developed by the Brainlab AG company was performed and evaluated on the transiliosacral screw fixation surgery, aiming at minimizing the surgical risks. However, this commercial navigation system is expensive and the lack of software expandability is obvious. As a result, the individual requirements of the surgeons cannot be met. Compared with some commercial visualization and medical image processing software, 3D Slicer (or just Slicer) is a free open source software platform for the community of computer-aided surgery, and it supports the development of extension modules. Although many researcher groups have presented the surgical navigation systems based on Slicer for various surgeries in the literature, their applications in percutaneous sacroiliac joint screw fixation are rarely reported.

In this contribution, a new loadable module ("SNS" module) based on Slicer was developed to achieve computer-aided navigation, aiming at improving the safety of percutaneous sacroiliac joint screw fixation surgery. The presented software module allows the calibration of surgical tools including "Pivot Calibration", "Axis Calibration of surgical drill" and "Surface Calibration of surgical saw", high-accuracy registration (point-based and surface matching), intra-operative motion tracking and virtual intra-operative CT imaging. The implementation and workflow of the designed Slicer module has been described in detail and validated through a cadaver experiment. With the support of other modules like "Editor", "Models", "OpenIGTLinkIF", "Fiducial Registration", etc., image segmentation, 3D-reconstruction, preoperative surgical planning, registration and intra-operative motion tracking can all be realized in Slicer. In addition, the "SNS" module can also be extended to various surgeries such as ear, nose, throat and oral implantology, and will be open-sourced to the global research community.

On the other hand, the Augmented Reality technology has great potential to apply to the computer-aided surgical navigation system. Some examples of AR-based surgical applications have been presented in the literature, for example, a hybrid tracking method for surgical augmented reality (University of Tubingen, Germany), an integral videography system (University of Tokyo, Japan), an alternative biopsy guidance system (University of Pittsburgh, America), an X-ray C-arm system (Technical University of Munich, Germany), etc. In addition, the calibration of AR device is also introduced in some reports. For instance, Falko Kellner (University of Kiel, Germany) et al. proposed a calibration approach with optical see-through head mounted displays to improve the average distance judgment of users in 2012, but, there is a significant underestimation of distances in the virtual environment [24]. Yakup Genc (Siemens Corporate Research Imaging and Visualization Department, America) et al. developed a method to calibrate stereoscopic optical see-through HMDs based on the 3D alignment of a target in the physical world with a virtual object in user's view [25]. However, the calibration algorithm was only validated on a video see-through system, and the researchers did not validate it for the optical see-through system. Stuart J. Gilson (Department of Physiology, United Kingdom) placed a camera inside an optical see-through HMD to take pictures simultaneously of tracked object and features in the HMD display for performing camera calibration [26]. In this study, a method for calibrating an optical see-through HMD is introduced and validated on an optical see-through system, and a surgical navigation system based on AR has been developed.

With the use of this system, including 3D-reconstruction, preoperative planning, registration, and calibration of HMD, the 3D virtual critical anatomical structures are aligned with the actual structures of patient in real-world scenario during the real-time motion tracking process. Therefore, some disadvantages of the traditional surgical navigation (For example, surgeon is no longer obliged to switch between the real operation scenario and computer screen) are overcome, and the safety, accuracy, and reliability of the surgery may be improved. The cadaver experiment validates the feasibility of AR-SNS. However, it is just a pilot study and still under development. Furthermore, some other experiments will be conducted to test the accuracy and efficiency of this system. The typical method is to measure the average distance deviations between the preoperative surgical planning trajectory and postoperative CT data. The researchers from Germany recently have compared the accuracy of a navigation system for oral implantology using either a head-mounted display or a monitor as a device for visualization. The results show that using of an HMD has no major disadvantages compared to the monitor setting [27].

ACKNOWLEDGMENTS

This study was supported by Natural Science Foundation of China (Grant No.: 81171429), Shanghai Pujiang Talent Program (Grant No.: 13PJD018) and Medical and Technological Joint Science Research Fund of Shanghai Jiao Tong University (Grant No.:YG2011ZD05 and YG2012MS18).

REFERENCES

[1] Cleary, K. and Peters, T. M., Image-guided interventions: Technology review and clinical applications. *Annu. Rev. Biomed. Eng.,* no.12, pp. 119-42, Apr. 2010.

[2] Hong, J., Matsumoto, N., Ouchida, R., Komune, S. and Hashizume, M., Medical navigation system for otologic surgery based on hybrid registration and virtual intraoperative computed tomography. *IEEE Trans. Biomed. Eng.,* vol. 56, no. 2, pp. 426-432, Feb. 2009.

[3] (2014, April 11). [Online]. Available: http://en.wikipedia.org/wiki /Computer-assisted_surgery.

[4] Behrendt, D., Mütze, M., Steinke, H., Koestler, M., Josten, C. and Böhme, J., Evaluation of 2D and 3D navigation for iliosacral screw fixation. Int. J. CARS, vol. 7, pp. 249-255, 2012.

[5] (2014, June 10). [Online]. Available: http://www.skullysystems.com/# home.

[6] Azuma, R., Baillot, Y., Behringer, R., Feiner, S., Julier, S. and MacIntyre. B., Recent advances in augmented reality. *IEEE Computer Graphics and Applications.* 21: 34-47, 2001.

[7] Yang, M. D., Chao, C. F., Huang, K. S., Lu, L. Y. and Chen, Y. P., Image-based 3D scene reconstruction and exploration in augmented reality. *Automation in Construction.* 33: 48-60, 2013.

[8] Navab, N., Traub, J., Sielhorst, T., Feuerstein, M. and Bichlmeier, C., Action- and workflow-driven augmented reality for computer-aided medical procedures. *IEEE Computer Society.* 27: 10-14, 2007.

[9] Liao, H., Dohi, T. and Iwahara, M., Improved viewing resolution of integral videography by use of rotated prism sheets. *Opt. Express.* 15: 4814-4822, 2007.

[10] Liao, H., Inomata, T., Sakuma, I. and Dohi, T., 3-D augmented reality for MRI-Guided surgery using integral videography autostereoscopic image overlay. *IEEE Trans. on Biomed. Eng.* 57: 1476-1486, 2010.

[11] Navab, N., Heining, S. M. and Traub, J., Camera augmented mobile C-arm (CAMC): calibration, accuracy study and clinical applications. *IEEE Trans. Med. Imaging.* 29: 1412-1423, 2010.

[12] Lorensen, W. E. and Cline, H. E., Marching cubes: A high resolution 3D surface construction algorithm. *ACM Computer Graphics*, vol. 21, pp. 38-44, 1987.

[13] Fitzpatrick, J. M., West, J. B. and Maurer, C. R., Predicting error in rigid body point-based registration. *IEEE Trans. Med. Imag.,* vol. 17, no. 5, pp. 694-702, Oct. 1998.

[14] West, J. B., Fitzpatrick, J. M., Toms, S. A., Maurer, C. R. and Maciunas, R. J., Fiducial point placement and the accuracy of point-based rigid body registration. *Neurosurgery*, vol.48, pp. 810-816, Apr. 2001.

[15] Claes, J., Koekelkoren, E., Wuyts, F. L., Claes, G. M. E., Van Den Hauwe, L. and Van de Heyning, P. H., Accuracy of computer navigation in ear, nose, throat surgery-The influence of matching strategy. *Otolaryngol. Head Neck Surg.*, vol. 126, pp. 1462-1466, Dec. 2000.

[16] Schicho, K., Figl, M., Seemanm, R., Donat, M., Pretterklieber, M. L., Birkfellner, W., Reichwein, A., Wanschitz, F., Kainberger, F., Bergmann, H., Wagner, A. and Ewers, R., Comparison of laser surface scanning and fiducial marker-based registration in frameless stereotaxy. *J. Neurosurg.*, vol. 106, pp. 704-709, Apr. 2007.

[17] Caversaccio, M., Zulliger, D., Bachler, R., Nolte, L. P. and Hausler, R., Practical aspects for optimal registration (matching) on the lateral skull base with an optical frameless computer-aided pointer system. *Amer. J. Otol.*, vol. 21, pp. 863-870, Nov. 2000.

[18] Chen, X. J., Lin, Y. P., Wu, Y. Q. and Wang, C. T., Real-time motion tracking in image-guided oral implantology. *Int. J. Med. Robotics Comput. Assist Surg.*, vol. 4, pp. 339-347, Sep. 2008.

[19] Cleary, K., Cheng, P., Enquobahrie, A. and Yaniv, Z., IGSTK: The Book. Signature Book Printing, Gaithersburg, Maryland, 2009.

[20] Maurer, C. R., Fitzpatrick, J. M., Wang, M. Y., Galloway, R. L., Maciunas, R. J. and Allen, G. S., Registration of head volume images using implantable fiducial markers. *IEEE Trans. Med. Imaging*, vol. 16, pp. 447-462, Aug. 1997.

[21] Chen, X. J., Ye, M., Lin, Y. P., Wu, Y. Q. and Wang, C. T., Image guided oral implantology and its application in the placement of zygoma

implants. *Computer Methods and Programs in Biomedicine*, vol. 93, pp. 162-173, 2009.

[22] (2013, June 14). [Online]. Available: http://www.slicer.org/slicerWiki /index.php/Documentation/Nightly/Modules/OpenIGTLinkIF.

[23] Besl, P. J. and Mckay, N. D., A method for registration of 3-D shapes. *IEEE Trans. Pattern Anal. Machine Intell.,* vol. 14, pp. 239-256, Feb. 1992.

[24] Kellner, F., Bolte, B., Bruder, G., Rautenberg, U., Steinicke, F., Lappe, M. and Koch, R., Geometric calibration of head-mounted displays and its effects on distance estimation. *IEEE. Trans. on Visualization and Computer Graphics.* 18: 589-596, 2012.

[25] Genc, Y., Sauer, F., Wenzel, F., Tuceryan, M. and Navab, N., Optical see-through HMD calibration: A stereo method validated with a video see-through system. *IEEE and ACM Int. Symposium on Augmented Reality.* 165-174, 2000.

[26] Gilson, S. J., Fitzgibbon, A. W. and Glennerster, A., Spatial calibration of an optical see-through head mounted display. *J. Neurosci Methods.* 173: 140-146, 2008.

[27] Vigh, B., Muller, S., Ristow, O., Deppe, H., Holdstock, S., Hollander, J. D., Navab, N., Steiner, T. and Hohlweg-Majert, B., The use of a head-mounted display in oral implantology: a feasibility study. *Int. J. CARS.* 9: 71-78, 2014.

In: Computer-Assisted Surgery
Editor: Xiaojun Chen

ISBN: 978-1-63463-811-1

Chapter 2

APPLICATION OF NAVIGATION SYSTEM IN BIMAXILLARY SURGERY

Sun Yi and Constantinus Politis*
Stomatology and Maxillofacial Surgery,
KU Leuven University, Leuven, Flanders, Belgium

ABSTRACT

Perioperative navigation is an upcoming tool in orthognathic surgery. This chapter contains two parts. The aim of this chapter is to evaluate the accuracy of image-guided maxillary positioning in the sagittal and vertical directions. 18 patients (12 males, 6 females) underwent bimaxillary surgery with the use of perioperative navigation. During Le Fort I osteotomy, the KolibriTM surgical navigation system was used to control movement of the maxilla at the edge of the central upper incisor in the sagittal (buccal surface) and vertical (incisal edge) direction. At one week after surgery, a postoperative lateral cephalogram was taken and was registered to the preoperative lateral cephalogram to identify the actual surgical movement of the maxilla. Student's two-tailed paired t-test was used to evaluate differences between the planned and actual surgical movement of the maxilla, which were 0.63 ± 0.50 mm ($p = 0.12$) in the sagittal direction and 0.57 ± 0.37 mm ($p = 0.45$) in the vertical direction.

* Correspondence to: Stomatology and Maxillofacial Surgery. KU Leuven University, Kapucijnenvoer 7 blok a-box 7001, 3000 Leuven. Email: constantinus.politis@uzleuven.be

Our findings show that the navigation system is a useful perioperative tool to control the surgical change of the maxilla in bimaxillary surgery.

Keywords: Perioperative navigation, anatomic landmark-based registration, accuracy of image-guided maxillary positioning

Precise positioning of the maxilla is an important determinant of the aesthetic and functional outcomes of orthognathic surgery. Bimaxillary surgery is usually performed in two phases to achieve proper positioning: the preoperative surgical planning and intermediate splint construction, followed by the precise positioning of the maxilla during surgery with the help of the pre-fabricated intermediate and final splints.

Previous studies have shown that a number of inaccuracies can occur during facebow registration, transferring the facebow data to the articulator, and model surgery to fabricate the intermediate splint. Several different methods have been introduced to improve the accuracy of the intermediate splint [1, 2, 5, 6, 16, 17, 25, 26]. Recently, the concept of computer-assisted virtual surgical planning has been introduced. Different methods have been developed to simulate the cut of the jaws, and to virtually place the upper and lower jaws into the desired position [4, 13, 23, 24, 27]. The digital intermediate splint and the final splint are then fabricated through CAD/CAM technology. These rapid prototyping splints have a high degree of accuracy compared to conventional manually fabricated splints [8].

The principle behind the surgical technique has not changed over the past twenty years. During bimaxillary surgery, when the maxilla is mobilized first, the vertical change of the maxilla can be controlled using an intraoral reference point (IRP) [10] or an extraoral reference point (ERP) [7, 9, 11, 15, 18, 19]. Both methods have been proven to have good accuracy in the vertical direction. Regarding the transversal plane , precision relies on the use of the intermediate splint to position the maxilla as planned. The mobility of the temporomandibular joint (TMJ) can potentially lead to inaccuracies, especially in the sagittal direction, and it is sometimes very difficult to achieve full control of, e.g., a multi-segmented maxilla in all dimensions. Therefore, even a good intermediate splint is not always sufficient to precisely position the maxilla in the sagittal direction. There is currently no simple perioperative tool that allows the surgeon to control the surgical change of the maxilla during the operation, especially in the sagittal direction.

Navigation systems are widely used in the operating room to improve surgical accuracy. Bell [3] previously reported the clinical outcome of image-guided orthognathic surgery; however, the accuracy of the surgery was not quantified. The purpose of this chapter is to evaluate the accuracy of image-guided maxillary repositioning in the sagittal and vertical directions.

1.1. Materials and Methods

18 patients (12 males, 6 females) underwent bimaxillary surgery with perioperative use of the Kolibri™ navigation system (Brainlab AG, Feldkirchen, Germany). A preoperative lateral cephalogram was obtained four weeks before the operation. Surgical treatment was planned based on cast model study, clinical examination and lateral cephalogram tracing. All patients were scheduled for a one-piece Le Fort I osteotomy with a bilateral sagittal split osteotomy (BSSO) of the lower jaw as a second step during the bimaxillary procedure. Wax bite registrations were taken with the teeth in centric relation, followed by facebow registration. Model surgery following the surgical treatment plan was performed on the ARH articulator (Dentatus, Spanga, Sweden). One week before surgery, an intermediate splint was manually fabricated, which was placed inside the patient's mouth on the evening before the operation to ensure that it correctly fit on the occlusal surface.

Each patient was scanned using a SkyView (Cefla dental, Imola, Italy) cone beam computed tomography (CBCT) scanner four weeks before the operation using the following parameters: 9-inch field of view and dentition mode. Each slice was composed of 512 × 512 pixels, and the voxel size was 0.3 × 0.3 × 0.3 mm. The DICOM (Digital Image Communications in Medicine) data was imported into the iPlan ENT 3.0.0 surgical planning software (Brainlab AG, Feldkirchen, Germany). In this program, the Frankfort horizontal plane (FHP) was orientated as the X-Y plane and the nasion perpendicular plane was orientated as the Y-Z plane. The following six anatomical landmarks were selected for point-based registration: the left and right infraorbital foramen, the anterior nasal spine, the tips of the left and right upper canines, and the mesial contact points of the left and right upper incisors (Figure 1). The prepared surgical planning was transferred to the navigation system via USB stick.

The navigation system was set up in a standard operating room. The preoperative CBCT images were displayed on the monitor of the navigation system. With the patient under general anesthesia, the reference star array was securely attached to the patient's skull with a fixation screw (Figure 2). At the beginning of the operation, an experienced surgeon performed patient-to-image registration, following the protocol described by Sun et al. [22]. After patient-to-image registration, when the tip of the VectorVision[2] Pointer (Brainlab AG, Feldkirchen, Germany) was placed on a specific anatomic landmark, the position of the pointer tip in the patient space was calculated automatically through the navigation system and transferred to the corresponding position in the preoperative CBCT image space. The position of the pointer tip was projected on the preoperative CBCT image as a green cross.

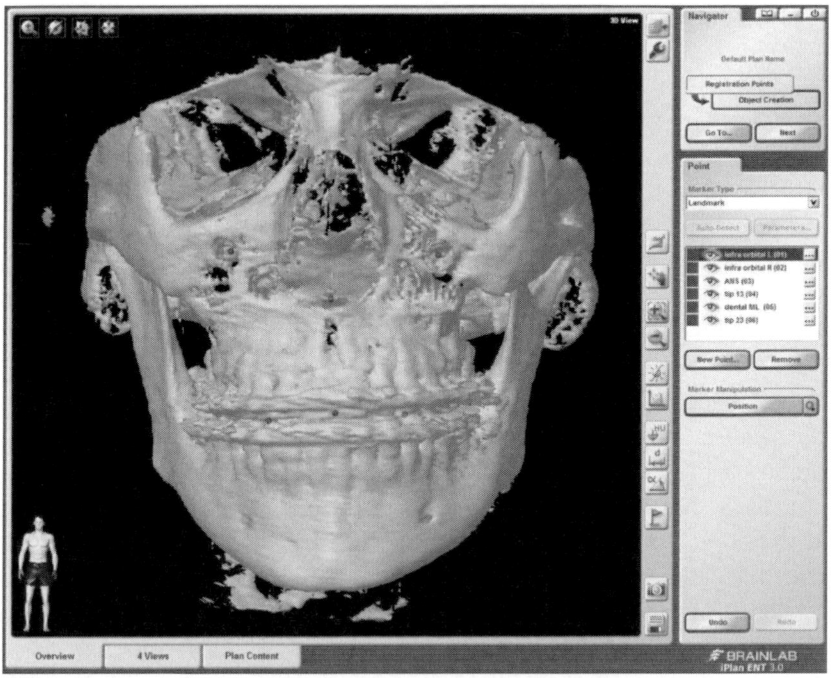

Figure 1. Six anatomical landmarks were indicated in the planning software (iPlan ENT 3.0.0): the left and right infraorbital foramen, the anterior nasal spine, the tips of the left and right upper canines, and the mesial contact point of the left and right upper incisors.

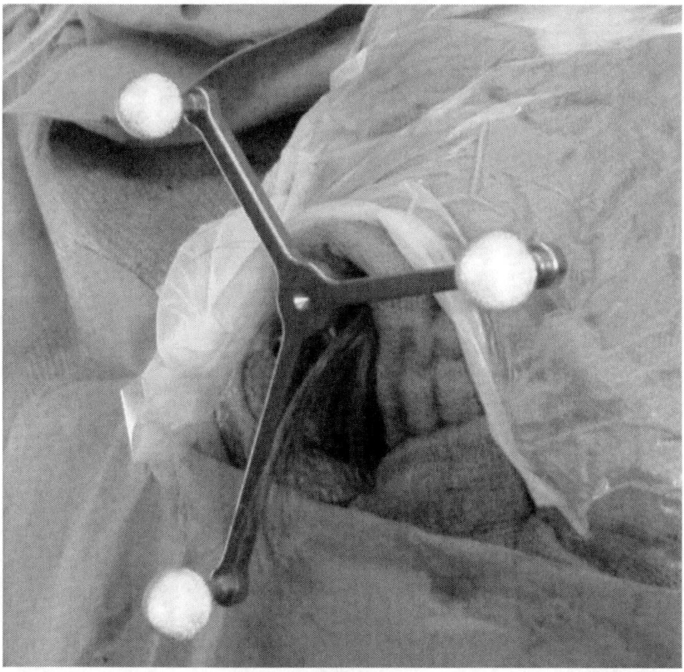

Figure 2. The reference star array was securely attached to the skull of the patient.

The VectorVision^2 Pointer was used to ensure the accuracy of the registration on the following anatomic points: the tips of the left and right upper canines and the upper incisors. The VectorVision^2 Pointer was also used to mark a reference point at the tip of the central upper incisor, which appeared as blue dot on the CBCT image in the navigation system. Registration was accepted if no discrepancy was observed between pointer position in the surgical field and the position of the green cross in the CBCT dataset.

A Tekka screw was inserted at the base of nose. After the down-fracture of the maxilla, intermaxillary fixation was applied using the intermediate splint to reposition the maxillary teeth in the desired occlusion. While the intermediate splint allowed the surgeon to place the maxilla at the desired position in the transversal and sagittal planes, the vertical position was dictated, not by the intermediate splint, but rather by manual intrusion or extrusion rotation on the condyle of the mandible. The vertical change of the maxilla was first controlled using a caliper by repeated measurement of the distance between the Tekka screw and the edge of the upper incisor before and after maxillary positioning.

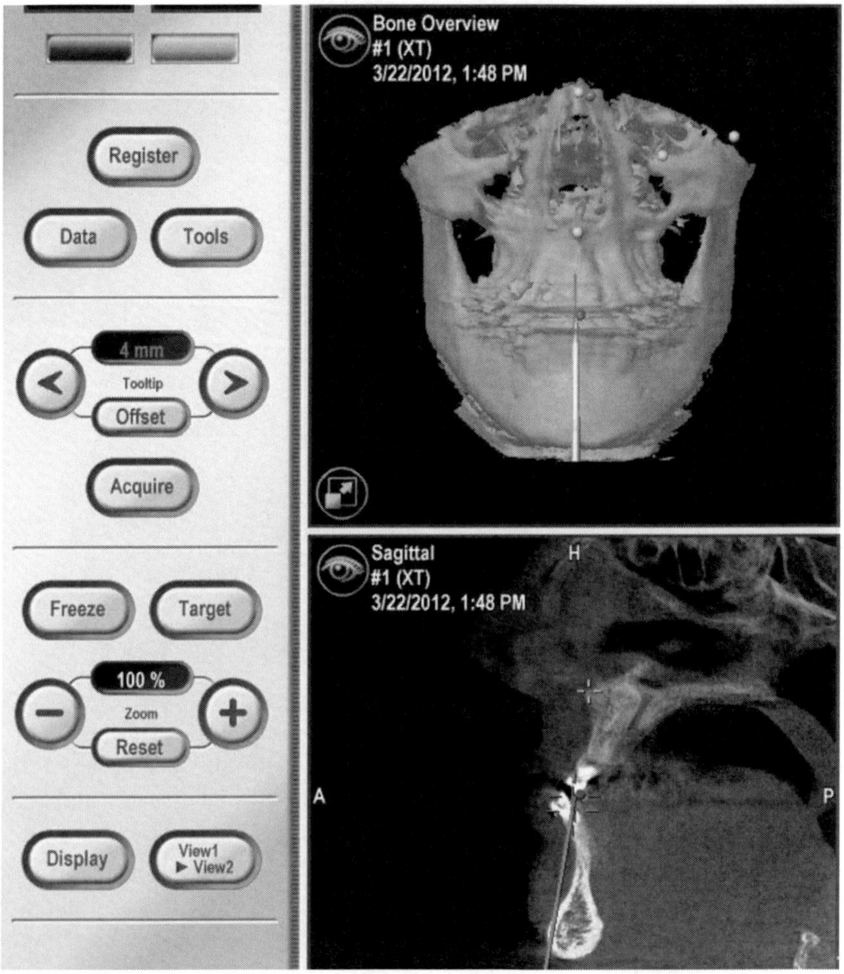

Figure 3. The blue point was acquired at the edge of the upper central incisor after the patient-to-image registration. After Le Fort I osteotomy, to measure the vertical movement of the maxilla using the navigation system, the pointer tip was physically positioned at the edge of the upper central incisor. The axis of the pointer was orientated perpendicular to the FHP. In this example, the pointer tip was projected on the preoperative CBCT image as green cross. The pointer offset was 4 mm along the vertical direction until it (red cross) reached the edge of the upper central incisor in the preoperative CBCT image. The figure illustrated that the surgical change in the vertical direction was 4mm. (*From* Sun Y, Luebbers HT, Agbaje JO, Lambrichts I, Politis C. The accuracy of image-guided navigation for maxillary positioning in bimaxillary surgery. J Craniofac Surg 2014;25(3):1095-9)

The VectorVision[2] Pointer was then used to check the vertical change at the edge of the upper central incisor. The pointer was physically positioned at the edge of the central incisor. The axis of the pointer was then orientated perpendicular to the FHP. On the preoperative CBCT image, coming from the green cross, which represented the pointer tip, an offset along the vertical direction was set until it (red cross) reached the edge of the upper central incisors (Figure 3).

The amount of the offset was noted as the surgical change in the vertical direction. The minimum offset was 1 mm. When there was a discrepancy between the vertical measurements from the caliper and the pointer, the measurement of the navigation system was preferred.

To check the surgical movement of the maxilla in the sagittal direction, the pointer was physically positioned at the edge of the central incisor. The axis of the pointer was then orientated parallel to the FHP. On the preoperative CBCT image, coming from the green cross, which represented the pointer tip, an offset along the sagittal direction was set until it (red cross) reached the edge of the upper central incisors (buccal surface) (Figure 4).

The amount of the offset was noted as the surgical change in the sagittal direction. The minimum offset was 1 mm. Since the sagittal position of the maxilla is also determined by the manual compression exerted on the condyle during maxillary repositioning over the intermaxillary fixation, small sagittal corrections could be made until the pointer indicated that the preplanned sagittal position of the upper incisor was reached. The maxilla was then held in the desired position and stabilized with four osteosynthesis plates, which were adapted to allow for passive placement without displacement of bone during fixation of the osteosynthesis screws. Once the upper jaw was stabilized, the navigation system was used to re-check the surgical movement in the sagittal and vertical directions at the edge of the upper central incisors. This final measurement from the navigation system was recorded for each patient.

At one week after surgery, a postoperative lateral cephalogram was obtained. Surgically unaffected structures of the skull base were used to superimpose the preoperative cephalogram tracing onto the postoperative lateral cephalogram image. The sagittal direction was defined by the preoperative FHP. The vertical direction was perpendicular to the FHP. The actual surgical movement at the edge of central incisor point of the maxilla was measured separately in the sagittal and vertical directions. These measurements were repeated four weeks later by the same observer. For each patient, the actual surgical movement was calculated over these two measurements.

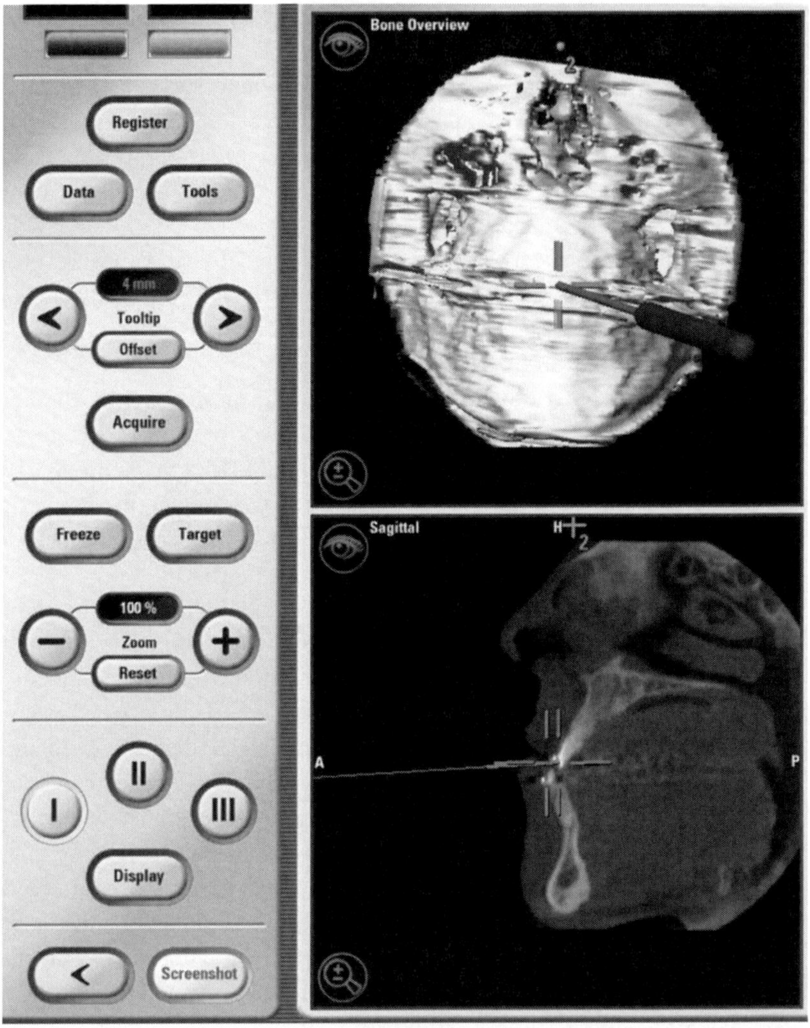

Figure 4. After Le Fort I osteotomy, to measure the sagittal movement of the maxilla using the navigation system, the pointer tip was physically positioned at the edge of the upper central incisor. The axis of the pointer was orientated parallel to the FHP. In this example, pointer tip was projected on the preoperative CBCT image as green cross. The pointer offset was 4 mm along the sagittal direction until it (red cross) reached the edge of the upper central incisor (buccal surface) in the preoperative CBCT image. The figure illustrated that the surgical change in the sagittal direction was 4mm. (*From* Sun Y, Luebbers HT, Agbaje JO, Lambrichts I, Politis C. The accuracy of image-guided navigation for maxillary positioning in bimaxillary surgery. J Craniofac Surg 2014; 25(3):1095-9)

Statistical analysis was performed using MedCalc (MedCalc Software bvba, Belgium). Student's two-tailed paired *t*-test was performed to determine intra-observer reliability; as well as to make comparisons between the planned and the actual surgical movement of the maxilla in the sagittal and vertical directions, and between the measurement results from the navigation system and the actual surgical movement in the sagittal and vertical directions. Differences were considered statistically significant if $p \leq 0.05$.

1.2. Results

The preoperative surgical planning included movement of 2 to 6.5 mm in the sagittal direction (defined as advancement/setback) and movement of −8.5 to 4.5 mm in the vertical direction (defined as intrusion/extrusion), with advancement and extrusion represented by movement in the positive direction.

Patient-to-image registration was successful and uneventful in all patients. Evaluation of intra-observer reliability revealed no significant differences between the two measurements based on cephalographic images: sagittal (p = 0.27) and vertical (p = 0.14). The absolute mean differences between the first and the second measurements were 0.14 mm and 0.16 mm in the sagittal and vertical directions, respectively. In the sagittal direction, the absolute mean difference between the planned and the actual surgical change was 0.63 ± 0.50 mm (0.1–2.1 mm; p = 0.12). The absolute mean difference between the measurement result from the navigation system and the actual surgical change was 0.47 ± 0.33 mm (0.1–1.27 mm; p = 0.19). The absolute mean difference between the preoperative surgical planning and the measurement result from the navigation system was 0.33 ± 0.45 mm (0–1 mm) (Table 1).

In the vertical direction, the difference between the measurement with the caliper and the measurement from the navigation system was more than 1 mm in two out of 18 patients. The absolute mean difference between the planned and the actual surgical change was 0.57 ± 0.37 mm (0–1.1 mm; p = 0.45). The absolute mean difference between the measurement result from the navigation system and the actual surgical change was 0.64 ± 0.41 (0–1.54 mm; p = 0.94). The absolute mean difference between the preoperative surgical planning and the measurement result from the navigation system was 0.17 ± 0.30 mm (0–1 mm) (Table 2).

Table 1. Distribution of the differences between the surgical treatment plan, measurement results from the navigation system, and actual surgical change at the edge of the upper central incisor in the sagittal direction (n = 18)

	Range (mm)				Absolute mean ± SD (range) in mm
	0–0.5	0–1	0–1.5	>1.5	
Planned - actual	10 (55.6%)	15 (83.3%)	17 (94.4%)	1 (5.6%)	0.63 ± 0.50 (0.1–2.1)
Navigation - actual	12 (66.7%)	16 (88.9%)	18 (100%)	0 (0%)	0.47 ± 0.33 (0.1–1.27)
Planned - navigation	13 (72.2%)	18 (100%)	18 (100%)	0 (0%)	0.33 ± 0.45 (0–1)

Table 2. Distribution of the differences between the surgical treatment plan, measurement results from the navigation system, and the actual surgical movement at the edge of the upper central incisor in the vertical direction (n = 18)

	Range (mm)				Absolute mean ± SD (range) in mm
	0–0.5	0–1	0–1.5	>1.5	
Planned - actual	8 (44.4%)	17 (94.4%)	18 (100%)	0 (0%)	0.57 ± 0.37 (0–1.1)
Navigation - actual	6 (33.3%)	17 (94.4%)	17 (94.4%)	1 (5.6%)	0.64 ± 0.41 (0–1.54)
Planned - navigation	17 (94.4%)	18 (100%)	18 (100%)	(0 %)	0.17 ± 0.30 (0–1)

1.3. Discussion

Successful orthognathic surgery requires repositioning the maxilla as precisely as possible in accordance with the preoperative surgical planning. The surgical accuracy at the anterior maxilla, especially at the incisor tip, is very important for aesthetic reasons, as small inaccuracies of the upper incisor position can affect the patient's satisfaction, particularly if they occur in the vertical position.

The ERP technique used to control the vertical change of maxillary repositioning is highly precise, with previous studies reporting maxillary positioning vertical deviations of between 0.37 and 1 mm [7, 11, 15, 18, 19]. In our study, the surgical change of the maxilla was controlled by the navigation system, and we observed a variation of 0.57 ± 0.37 mm in the vertical direction between the preoperative surgical plan and the actual surgical movement, which was comparable to previous studies using the ERP method.

A most recent study by Gil et al. [9] reported an even better accuracy of 0.3 ± 0.20 mm in the vertical direction using medial canthal region as an ERP. In another study [10], where an improved internal reference point (IRP) technique was applied, 81% of the patients showed a variation of within 0.4 mm in the vertical direction.

There is typically a larger deviation in the sagittal direction. Polido et al. [19] reported that the average deviation of sagittal maxillary positioning was about 1.7 mm, which was greater than the deviation in the vertical positioning (1 mm). Ong et al. [15] reported a mean difference of 0.85 mm between the planned and the actual surgical movement in the sagittal direction. Similarly, Kretschmer et al. [11] found a median difference of 1 mm between the planned and the actual surgical movement in the sagittal direction. Deviation in the sagittal direction is likely due to several sources of error: errors associated with the facebow recording, transferring face bow to the articulator, model surgery to fabricate the intermediate splint and the mobility of the TMJ [20, 28]. The present study showed that image guidance improved the deviation in the sagittal direction to a mean of 0.63 mm (0.1–2.1 mm). Omura et al. [14] described another method of joint fixation with positioning plates to improve the accuracy of the maxillary positioning; however, this technique required an additional surgical procedure and it is difficult to manage during surgery. Kretschmer et al. [11] mentioned the clinical outcome of a similar technique, in which 75.2% of the deviations were within 1 mm in both the sagittal and vertical directions. In our study, 83.3% of the patients showed a variation of within 1 mm between the planned and the actual movement of the maxilla in the sagittal direction. This finding was comparable to those mentioned by Kretschmer et al. [11] and was better than those reported by Polido et al. [19] (39%) and Stanchina et al. [21] (65%).

In our study, the average deviations between the measurement results from the navigation system and the actual surgical movement were within 0.65 mm in both the sagittal and vertical directions. There were no significant differences between the measurement results of the navigation system and the actual surgical movements in both the sagittal and vertical directions. These findings prove that the navigation system can directly assess the surgical movement of the maxilla in the operating room, and thus has the potential to eliminate the errors associated with facebow recording, transferring face bow to the articulator, model surgery to fabricate the intermediate splint and the mobility of the TMJ.

It must be noted that image-guided surgery can introduce additional errors. Firstly, the navigation system only reports the Euclidian distance between the tip position of the pointer in the world space and the target label in the imaging space. This direct measurement provides no clinically relevant information, it is more important to know the surgical change in sagittal/vertical direction respectively. To identify the surgical change in the sagittal direction, it is necessary to orientate the axis of the pointer parallel to the FHP. Similarly, to evaluate the vertical change of the maxilla, the axis of the pointer needs to be orientated perpendicular to the FHP. Because of the limited space in the oral cavity, it is almost impossible to perfectly measure the sagittal and vertical changes through the pointer, especially in the posterior regions of the maxilla. Additionally, during the operation, the minimum offset unit of the pointer is 1 mm. The surgeon can only estimate the surgical change to up to half of the minimum offset unit, meaning that the maximum accuracy of the measurement is 0.5 mm.

Human-related errors can occur in image-guided surgery, because it is difficult to keep the maxilla stable during maxilla fixation. Even under the guidance of the navigation system, it is difficult to avoid maxillary positioning errors during fixation of the osteosynthesis plates when eccentric drilling occurs or if the plates are not perfectly adapted to the bone in a passive way. Such error may reduce the accuracy of maxillary positioning in the sagittal direction. In our study, the maximum difference between the preoperative planning and the final measurement from the navigation system was within 1 mm.

Finally, the accuracy of the image-guided surgery is mainly defined by the target registration error (TRE). In our study, six anatomic landmarks were selected for patient-to-image registration, and we found maximum differences between the measurement results from the navigation system and the actual surgical movement of 1.27 mm and 1.54 mm in the sagittal and vertical directions, respectively. Sun et al. [22] used this method in an *in vitro* study with the same anatomic landmarks selected for paired point-based registration; similar to our findings, they found the mean TRE in the region of the maxilla to be 0.93 ± 0.31 mm, and the maximum TRE observed was 1.6 mm in the region of frontal maxilla. The TRE is one factor that limits the accuracy of image-guided surgery. In an ideal situation where physical error sources can be eliminated, the navigation system can give the surgeon confidence that the deviation between the planned and the actual surgical movement can be controlled within the range of the maximum TRE. To improve the accuracy of maxillary repositioning, other image registration techniques could be applied to diminish the TRE, e.g., template-based registration or fiducial screws can be inserted in the maxilla for point-based registration. Luebbers et al. [12] reported a maximum TRE of 0.9 mm in the periorbital region using a maxillary splint with only two fiducial screws inserted percutaneously on the lateral orbital rim. This registration technique is the most accurate among all previously studied techniques; however, additional surgical work is required and the procedure causes pain and discomfort to the patient.

The following issues should be considered when performing image-guided surgery: the set-up and use of the image-guided navigation system added 30–45 minutes to the surgical treatment time. The navigation star array is fixed on the skull and could possibly cause infection after the operation, although this seems unlikely.

1.4. Conclusion

In conclusion, our study demonstrates that intraoperative computer navigation combined with the use of intermediate splint is a useful additional tool for controlling the surgical change of the maxilla in bimaxillary surgery, enabling precise positioning of the maxilla during bimaxillary surgery. Overall, we find that a navigation system might be helpful for controlling the final surgical outcome during the operation, especially for non-experienced surgeons.

References

[1] Akram, A., Collin, J., Postlethwaite, K., Sweeney, G., Planned to perfection? Use of the model repositioning instrument to plan maxillary movements for orthognathic surgery. *Orthodontics (Chic.)* 12:130-133, 2011.

[2] Anwar, M., Harris, M., Model surgery for orthognathic planning. *Br J Oral Maxillofac Surg* 28:393-397, 1990.

[3] Bell, R. B., Computer planning and intraoperative navigation in orthognathic surgery. *J Oral Maxillofac Surg* 69:592-605, 2011.

[4] Choi, J. Y., Hwang, J. M., Baek, S. H., Virtual model surgery and wafer fabrication using 2-dimensional cephalograms, 3-dimensional virtual dental models, and stereolithographic technology. *Oral Surg Oral Med Oral Pathol Oral Radiol* 113:193-200, 2012.

[5] Cottrell, D. A., Wolford, L. M., Altered orthognathic surgical sequencing and a modified approach to model surgery. *J Oral Maxillofac Surg* 52:1010-1021, 1994.

[6] Ellis, E., 3rd, Accuracy of model surgery: evaluation of an old technique and introduction of a new one. *J Oral Maxillofac Surg* 48:1161-1167, 1990.

[7] Ferguson, J. W., Luyk, N. H., Control of vertical dimension during maxillary orthognathic surgery. A clinical trial comparing internal and external fixed reference points. *J Craniomaxillofac Surg* 20:333-336, 1992.

[8] Gateno, J., Xia, J., Teichgraeber, J. F., Rosen, A., Hultgren, B., Vadnais, T., The precision of computer-generated surgical splints. *J Oral Maxillofac Surg* 61:814-817, 2003.

[9] Gil, J. N., Campos, F. E., Claus, J. D., Gil, L. F., Marin, C., de Freitas S. F., Medial canthal region as an external reference point in orthognathic surgery. *J Oral Maxillofac Surg* 69:352-355, 2011.

[10] Gil, J. N., Claus, J. D., Manfro, R., Lima, S. M., Predictability of maxillary repositioning during bimaxillary surgery: accuracy of a new technique. *Int J Oral Maxillofac Surg* 36:296-300, 2007.

[11] Kretschmer, W. B., Zoder, W., Baciut, G., Baciut, M., Wangerin, K., Accuracy of maxillary positioning in bimaxillary surgery. *Br J Oral Maxillofac Surg* 47:446-449, 2009.

[12] Luebbers, H. T., Messmer, P., Obwegeser, J. A., Zwahlen, R. A., Kikinis, R., Graetz, K. W., Matthews, F., Comparison of different

registration methods for surgical navigation in cranio-maxillofacial surgery. *J Craniomaxillofac Surg* 36:109-116, 2008.

[13] Metzger, M. C., Hohlweg-Majert, B., Schwarz, U., Teschner, M., Hammer, B., Schmelzeisen, R., Manufacturing splints for orthognathic surgery using a three-dimensional printer. *Oral Surg Oral Med Oral Pathol Oral Radiol Endod* 105:e1-7, 2008.

[14] Omura, S., Kimizuka, S., Iwai, T., Tohnai, I., An accurate maxillary superior repositioning technique without intraoperative measurement in bimaxillary orthognathic surgery. *Int J Oral Maxillofac Surg* 41:949-951, 2012.

[15] Ong, T. K., Banks, R. J., Hildreth, A. J., Surgical accuracy in Le Fort I maxillary osteotomies. *Br J Oral Maxillofac Surg* 39:96-102, 2001.

[16] Paul, P. E., Barbenel, J. C., Walker, F. S., Khambay, B. S., Moos, K. F., Ayoub, A. F., Evaluation of an improved orthognathic articulator system. 2. Accuracy of occlusal wafers. *Int J Oral Maxillofac Surg* 41:155-159, 2012a.

[17] Paul, P. E., Barbenel, J. C., Walker, F. S., Khambay, B. S., Moos, K. F., Ayoub, A. F., Evaluation of an improved orthognathic articulator system: 1. Accuracy of cast orientation. *Int J Oral Maxillofac Surg* 41:150-154, 2012b.

[18] Perkins, S. J., Newhouse, R. F., Bach, D. E., A modified Boley gauge for accurate measurement during maxillary osteotomies. *J Oral Maxillofac Surg* 50:1018-1019, 1992.

[19] Polido, W. D., Ellis, E., 3rd, Sinn, D. P., An assessment of the predictability of maxillary repositioning. *Int J Oral Maxillofac Surg* 20:349-352, 1991.

[20] Sharifi, A., Jones, R., Ayoub, A., Moos, K., Walker, F., Khambay, B., McHugh, S., How accurate is model planning for orthognathic surgery? *Int J Oral Maxillofac Surg* 37:1089-1093, 2008.

[21] Stanchina, R., Ellis, E., 3rd, Gallo, W. J., Fonseca, R. J., A comparison of two measures for repositioning the maxilla during orthognathic surgery. *Int J Adult Orthodon Orthognath Surg* 3:149-154, 1988.

[22] Sun, Y., Luebbers, H. T., Agbaje, J. O., Schepers, S., Vrielinck, L., Lambrichts, I., Politis, C., Validation of anatomical landmarks-based registration for image-guided surgery: an in-vitro study. *J Craniomaxillofac Surg* 41:522-526, 2013.

[23] Swennen, G. R., Mollemans, W., De Clercq, C., Abeloos, J., Lamoral, P., Lippens, F., Neyt, N., Casselman, J., Schutyser, F., A cone-beam computed tomography triple scan procedure to obtain a three-

dimensional augmented virtual skull model appropriate for orthognathic surgery planning. *J Craniofac Surg* 20:297-307, 2009.

[24] Tsuji, M., Noguchi, N., Shigematsu, M., Yamashita, Y., Ihara, K., Shikimori, M., Goto, M., A new navigation system based on cephalograms and dental casts for oral and maxillofacial surgery. *Int J Oral Maxillofac Surg* 35:828-836, 2006.

[25] Walker, F., Ayoub, A. F., Moos, K. F., Barbenel, J., Face bow and articulator for planning orthognathic surgery: 1 face bow. *Br J Oral Maxillofac Surg* 46:567-572, 2008a.

[26] Walker, F., Ayoub, A. F., Moos, K. F., Barbenel, J., Face bow and articulator for planning orthognathic surgery: 2 articulator. *Br J Oral Maxillofac Surg* 46:573-578, 2008b.

[27] Xia, J. J., Gateno, J., Teichgraeber, J. F., New clinical protocol to evaluate craniomaxillofacial deformity and plan surgical correction. *J Oral Maxillofac Surg* 67:2093-2106, 2009.

[28] Zizelmann, C., Hammer, B., Gellrich, N. C., Schwestka-Polly, R., Rana, M., Bucher, P., An evaluation of face-bow transfer for the planning of orthognathic surgery. *J Oral Maxillofac Surg* 70:1944-1950, 2012.

In: Computer-Assisted Surgery
Editor: Xiaojun Chen ISBN: 978-1-63463-811-1

Chapter 3

COMPUTER-ASSISTED MINIMALLY INVASIVE SURGERY: IMAGE-GUIDED INTERVENTIONS AND ROBOTIC SURGERY

Francisco M. Sánchez Margallo *
and Juan A. Sánchez Margallo
Jesús Usón Minimally Invasive Surgery Centre, Cáceres, Spain

ABSTRACT

Laparoscopic surgery represents one of the main evolutions of surgical techniques. However, this leads to some challenges that can be reduced through computer technology. This chapter presents a review of the state of the art of current methods for computer-assisted in laparoscopic surgery. Surgical navigation systems have the potential to improve information on the exact place of key anatomical structures such as vessels and tumors within the surgical field. With the support of navigation systems surgeons can potentially improve clinical outcomes of image-guided interventions. The use of image guidance methods such as augmented reality and near infrared fluorescence enhances visual information to supplement the two-dimensional imaging and the absence of tactile feedback in laparoscopic surgery. In the field of robotic surgery, robotic systems enable surgeons to perform advanced laparoscopic procedures with greater visualization and dexterity than traditional

* Correspondence to: Minimally Invasive Surgery Centre Jesús Usón. Ctra. N-521 Km 41,8; 10181 Cáceres, Spain. msanchez@ccmijesususon.com; Telephone: +34 927181032.

laparoscopic technology. Image-guided robots can be inserted into the patient's body by using real-time feedback from different imaging techniques. Recent developments in minimally invasive techniques have led to laparoendoscopic single-site surgery (LESS), which has a great potential in patient outcomes but remains technically challenging. Several robotic-assisted systems have been applied to single-site surgery to deal with these limitations. This has resulted in a new kind of surgery, robotic LESS or R-LESS. This work gives an overview of current developments in image-guided laparoscopic interventions regarding navigation systems and image guidance methods, as well as in new systems and applications of robotic surgery, especially in novel surgical techniques such as LESS and NOTES.

Keywords: Laparoscopic surgery, image-guided interventions, augmented reality, Rrobotic surgery

ABBREVIATIONS

5-ALA	5-aminolevulinic acid
AESOP	Automated Endoscopic System for Optimal Positioning
AR	Augmented reality
CAS	Computer-assisted surgery
CT	Computed tomography
DARPA	Defense Advanced Research Projects Agency
DOF	Degrees of freedom
FDA	Food and Drug Administration
ICG	Indocyanine green
IGS	Image-guided surgery
LESS	Laparo-endoscopic single-site surgery
MDCT	Multiple detector computed tomography
MIS	Minimally invasive surgery
MRI	Magnetic resonance imaging
NASA	National Aeronautics and Space Administration
NIRF	Near-infrared fluorescence
NOTES	Natural orifice transluminal endoscopic surgery
NSF	National Science Foundation
PDD	Photodynamic diagnostic
PpIX	Protoporphyrin IX

PUMA	Programmable Universal Machine for Assembly
RAL	Robotic-assisted laparoscopic
SPS	Surgical planning system
SRI	Stanford Research Institute
TEM	Transanal endoscopic microsurgery
TRUS	Transrectal ultrasound
US	Ultrasound
UVA	Ultraviolet A
VR	Virtual reality

1. INTRODUCTION

The introduction of minimally invasive surgery (MIS) has been one of the greatest advances in the surgical field in recent times. This kind of surgery tries to reduce the invasiveness for the patients, providing them with several benefits such as reduction of tissue trauma and postoperative pain, better aesthetic results, and less operative periods with the consequence reduction of the healthcare costs. These benefits have made these surgical techniques the focus of attention and the choice in many surgical procedures, which usually have been performed by open surgery. However, they have some limitations that should be addressed. In minimally invasive procedures the depth perception is lost, and surgeons have to perform the intervention using a two-dimensional (2D) interpretation of the surgical field. Besides, they have to use new surgical instruments that in most cases limit their surgical skills and hamper the ergonomic conditions during surgery. All the previous restrictions entail a steep learning curve for the surgeon.

Continuous advances in computer science make computer-assisted surgery (CAS) a new powerful way for addressing some of the aforementioned limitations, increasing and expanding surgeon's perceptions. The broad range of CAS represents the integration of computer technology in surgical procedures for presurgical planning, surgical guiding as well as surgical manipulation. Within the field of CAS, image-guided surgery (IGS) and surgical robots are the most challenging fields. Image-guided surgery provides surgeons with tools to apply preoperative information from the patient during the surgical performance as well as the possibility of preoperative planning. This allows the surgeon to determine the best way to tackle an operation and to treat a disease, and later use this information as support during the course of the intervention. Similarly, advances in robot technology have enabled the development of robotic surgical systems and devices for surgical assistance. These systems are created as tools to solve certain technical difficulties during the performance of some MIS techniques, providing three-dimensional (3D) view of the surgical field, improvement of the surgical instruments, increased surgical skills, improving ergonomics, and even providing tactile feedback during surgery. The objective of this chapter is to review the history and current status of computer-assisted in MIS. The chapter is organized into two main sections, which are focused on IGS and robotic-assisted surgery, as main components of CAS.

2. Image-Guided Surgery

In order to cope with some of the limitations in MIS and guide the surgeon during a surgical procedure, systems for IGS have been developed. The lack of tactile feedback and 3D sensation in video-assisted surgery accelerated the need for these systems. In addition, for the human eye, several pathologies, such as the presence of non-superficial tumors, are not easily distinguishable from surrounding normal tissue. This make, in some occasions, decision making during surgery a very difficult process. During IGS preoperative imaging data is used in conjunction with images from the operative field to improve the localization and targeting of pathologies, as well as monitor and control treatments. Several advanced in imaging technologies are used for IGS such as magnetic resonance imaging (MRI), computed tomography (CT), and even positron emission tomography (PET), which replace or complement direct visualization. The combination of tracking technologies for recording the position of the patient and the surgical instruments with preoperative and intraoperative images provides a comprehensive assistance tool for guiding any MIS intervention. Image-guided procedures are substantially less invasive than traditional surgery. Image-guided technology allows for more precise and accurate procedures and surgeons can decide the best approach to address a specific disease before the intervention, which may reduce the operating times as well as the number of surgical ports needed.

In general, there are some common steps followed to carry out an image-guided surgical intervention [1,2]. Initially, the patient undergoes diagnostic imaging, in most cases CT or MRI. These images are then converted and processed into a 3D model of the patient's anatomy. This information is subsequently used for preoperative surgical planning and/or intraoperative surgical decision making. During the operation, the virtual model and the surgical planning are used as a guide for navigating into the patient anatomy. During this process, the surgical instruments are tracked and mapped with respect to the virtual model to increase the accuracy during the procedure and minimize damage to normal tissues. This 3D navigation helps a surgeon to better visualize and understand the internal anatomy of the patient during each surgical step.

2.1. Components of Image-guided Surgery

IGS integrates three major technologies: imaging, tracking, registration and visualization technologies. Each of these components will be described in more detail below.

2.1.1. Image Acquisition and Rendering

The fundamental basis of IGS is diagnostic imaging, and its progress primarily depends on technological advances in this field. No unique imaging system is exclusively used for diagnostic imaging, many different imaging modalities have been used for IGS, including ultrasound (US), MR and X-Ray imaging. All diagnostic imaging modalities have been used to guide procedures with or without some modification or adjustment. However, most image-guided navigation systems used CT or MRI systems. This is because they can provide a good quality 3D map of the anatomy, especially in the case of CT imaging. While most image-guided navigation systems are based on preoperative imaging, there is an increasing interest in using intraoperative imaging for navigation [3].

Once diagnostic imaging data of the patient has been recorded, this information needs to be processed. The goal of medical image processing is to extract quantitative information from the diagnostic images to better diagnose, localize, monitor, and treat surgical pathologies. Currently there are a large number of software tools to delineate, reconstruct and visualize patient organs and pathologies in 3D models obtained from medical imaging before surgery such as Myrian® from Intrasense, Ziostation® from Ziosoft, Synapse® Vincent from Fujinon, Iqqa® Liver from Edda Technology, Scout® Liver from Pathfinder, among others.

One of the main steps in image processing is the image segmentation. This is defined as structuring an image into different regions that are identified by signal intensities, textures, lines, or shapes. The resulting virtual model is defined by the different relevant anatomical structures that will take part during the surgical intervention [3]. Medical image segmentation is a challenging process. In diagnostic images not all the anatomical structures of interest are homogeneous and clearly separable from the surroundings. In some cases their grayscale value is not constant, and strong edges may not be present around borders. Additionally, image segmentation algorithms may not work well in the presence of poor image contrast, significant noise, and unclear anatomical boundaries. For this reason, in certain cases it is needed the intervention of an expert human operator to guide the process, which could be tedious and prone to error. Image segmentation is a fundamental step to support the surgical treatment of tumors or in case some critical anatomical structures should be avoided during the surgical intervention.

2.1.2. Tracking Technologies

In IGS it is crucial to record the 3D position and orientation of both the patient and the surgical instruments during the intervention. These positions will be mapped later on with the 3D model obtained from preoperative imaging (registration process), to precisely visualize the instrument motion with respect to the surrounding anatomical structures. Surgical navigation systems provide surgeons with a better visualization of the anatomical structures inside the body in relation to the actual position of surgical instruments, minimizing damage of surrounding health tissues.

Currently there are different tracking technologies that are commonly used for IGS such as optical videometric (Figure 1), optical active and passive infrared, and electromagnetic [4]. Among them, optical tracking systems are the most used. They are generally highly spatially accurate (more precise than 1 mm), but suffer from the line-of-sight restrictions between the tracking device and the object to be tracked and have some limitations to track flexible instruments. Electromagnetic tracking systems do not have this line-of-sight constraint and are capable of tracking flexible objects inside the body such as catheters and the instrument tip [5].

2.1.3. Registration

Registration is another essential component for IGS; with this process the real patient and the image-based model (virtual model) are co-registered in the same reference frame. The simplest registration method is to manually match a paired-point landmark, such as the umbilicus or a nipple, between the actual organ and the overlaying image [6]. In the most common clinical scenario, radiopaque markers are attached on the patient's skin to be registered in the preoperative CT or MRI studies. Although this method is useful when superimposed on skin or bone, it is not sufficient for complex soft intraabdominal organs (non-rigid registration).

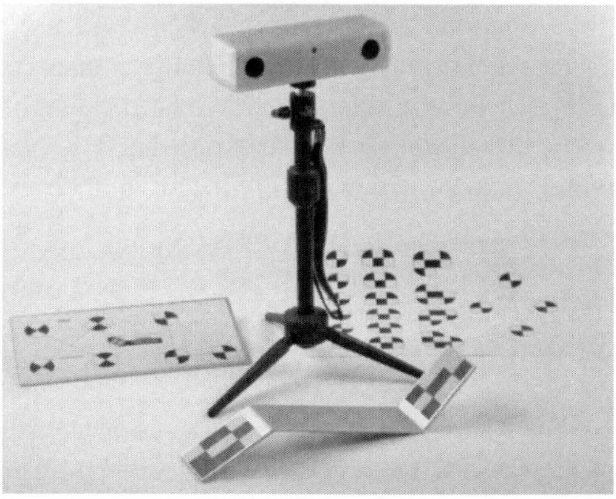

Figure 1. Videometric tracker with pattern-marked markers (Claron Technology Inc., Toronto, ON, Canada).

Registration can be broadly classified into two types: rigid registration or non-rigid registration [3]. Image registration is rigid when images are assumed to be solid and only need rotation and/or translation to be matched with each other. In commercial IGS, only rigid registration is used [4]. However, most of the anatomical structures presented in MIS are not rigid, and therefore deformations of these structures during surgery require the application of non-rigid registration algorithms, updating the anatomical changes in the intraoperative images [7,8]. Imaging data acquired by US and intraoperative CT have been specially utilized in cases requiring renewed real-time data for intraoperative deformation [9,10].

2.1.4. Visualization

The visualization techniques used to display the results during IGS can be categorized into three main types: projected images, additional monitor or transparent monitor [11,12]. The first method consists of projecting the virtual model directly onto the patient or the target organ [6]. However, in this visualization method the projector light beam may be interrupted by the surgical staff or equipment. Moreover, image deformations can occur when the images are projected onto irregular surfaces. The second method, which is the most used, makes use of an additional monitor to display the virtual model and additional information, in which the typical visualization is a four-quadrant presentation that usually consists of three orthogonal 2D images and a 3D rendering. The third method uses a transparent monitor or plate between the target organ and the surgeon's line of vision. In this case, the virtual model is superimposed on the actual real view through the transparent surface [13]. Additionally, there is a hybrid solution, which is the use of a video head-mounted display. In this case, the images from the IGS are displayed on a small video monitor mounted in front of one or both eyes using a head-mounted video camera.

2.2. Surgical Planning Systems

Surgical planning systems (SPS) use the 3D virtual models of a patient to develop a treatment plan and predefine the surgical steps. The 3D models of the patients are usually obtained from their CT or MRI preoperative imaging. These planning systems allow surgeons to interact with the virtual model of the patient, so that they can understand more in depth his/her anatomy and define the best operative strategy. SPS are excellent tools for assessing the patient's pathology and for preoperative decision-making (Figure 2). Preoperative surgical planning may improve the efficiency of MIS procedures thanks to better learning of patient anatomy and real preoperative training [14]. Therefore, using SPS surgeons can establish an improved diagnosis and a better planning of the best-suited therapy for each surgical case [15]. However, apart from all these positive implications, one limitation of these systems is the surgeon's learning curve.

Some of the features that typically include SPS are semi-automated or automated segmentation of relevant anatomical structures, identification of the lesion margins, accurate 3D model generation from the segmented data, selective visualization and transparency transforms [15,16]. These systems are particularly important for procedures where surgeons will be working close to nerves or vulnerable anatomical structures that could lead to significant consequences during surgery. The next step will be to transfer the previous surgical planning to the patient by means of a surgical navigation system.

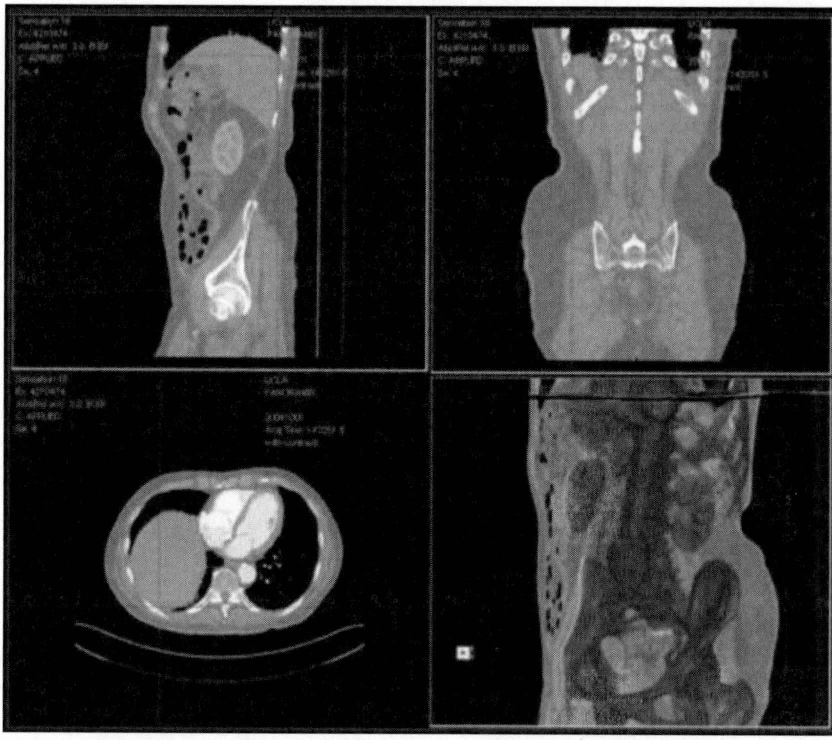

Figure 2. Example of a surgical planning system for intraabdominal surgery.

2.3. Surgical Navigation Systems

Surgical navigation systems (SNS), in which patient's preoperative information is used during the surgical intervention as a surgical decision-making tool, has been clinically applied in many fields to improve the safety, accuracy, and efficiency of surgeries. In MIS, due to surgeon has less visual and tactile perception than in open surgery, image assistance may be increasingly helpful for 3D understanding of the surgical target. The main aim of SNS is to specifically target an anatomical structure during surgery in safer and less invasive ways. Commercial based SNS are most widely used in neurosurgery [17], otolaryngology [18], and orthopedics [19], in which the target organs are assumed to be rigid and to have a constant spatial relationship to anatomical landmarks [20,21]. In more recent works, image-guided navigation has been extended to soft tissue applications like the liver and other abdominal organs [22,23]. However, the use of these systems in abdominal surgery is still a challenging task.

The basic setup of a SNS consists of a preoperative image data, a tracking system, a computer platform with screen, and the respective navigation software [4]. Navigation in general uses preoperative image data for example form CT or MRI images, which are used for navigation in the OR (image acquisition). Before surgery, surgical strategy, steps, paths for the surgical instruments, and objects and areas of interest may be planned using a virtual model obtained from the preoperative images (planning). During surgery, the preoperative image data need to be matched to the current patient position by means of the tracking systems (registration). If required, the surgeon may obtain additional images during the surgery and register and include them in the running navigation.

2.3.1. Augmented Reality

The use of SNS allows surgeons to see patient's anatomical structures obtained from preoperative imaging or a prior surgical planning. However, when this information is displayed on an independent monitor, a distance between this visual information and the actual patient surgical field is created. In order to eliminate this gap, augmented reality (AR) applied to the surgical navigation is developed. Navigation surgery using AR consists in superimposing the preoperative 3D patient modeling onto the real intraoperative view of the patient [14,24], thus augmenting the real view with virtual information. AR has the potential to enhance the understanding of the pathological and surrounding anatomy during surgery by means of projecting the 3D model of the interested region. From the patient's medical images such as US, CT or MRI, AR techniques increase the surgeon's intraoperative vision by providing a virtual transparency of the patient [14]. Fine definition of dissection planes, resection margins and avoidance of injury to invisible structures are substantial applications of AR in abdominal surgery [9,25].

AR is based on two major processes: 3D modeling and visualization of anatomical or pathological structures appearing in the medical image, and the registration of this visualization onto the real patient [14]. The preoperative reconstructed images are registered with anatomic landmarks or artificial markers on the patient and then these images are tracked with regard to the patient's position, intraoperative images, as well as instruments and camera movements. Best preoperative imaging modalities are usually offered by CT and MRI, but one of the main constraints is that surgical anatomy changes drastically during surgery. Therefore, one of the most challenging aspects of

AR applied to surgery is to register and merge preoperative and intraoperative images, where tracking devices are the principal protagonists in order to relate these two concepts [26]. Tracking devices link spatial information from imaging modalities, anatomical landmarks, instruments, by representing these in one common coordinate system and establishing a simple registration [26,27]. Among intraoperative imaging, US has been the most widely used image acquisition.

Surgical navigation based on AR could be defined as the next step in IGS. However, this imaging technique remains currently limited by the registration of organs deformation during surgery, the lack of studies to prove its usefulness, and the portability and cost of the required equipment [11]. The use of AR navigations systems has been extensively used in neurosurgery, otolaryngology, orthopedics, and maxillofacial surgery [21]. These surgeries allow for precise registration thanks to rigid organs and bone structures. In the case of abdominal surgery the use of AR is more challenging. One of the main problems is the need to provide a real-time updating of the changes that occur in intraabdominal structures caused by breathing, heartbeat, patient movement and interactions by the surgeons. In order to deal with these problems, soft tissue navigation methods are being developed.

Marescaux et al. [28] reported the first use of an AR-assisted intervention for adrenalectomy without a tracking system for the laparoscope. The virtual model was obtained from a CT scan of the patient. Then, segmentation of the intraabdominal organs and 3D reconstruction of the lesion were performed. During surgery, an operator adapted manually the virtual model to the real laparoscopic images by using 7 different visible landmarks on the skin (right costal margin and 3 trocar sites) and inside the abdomen (inferior vena cava and 2 laparoscopic tools). These AR images were displayed on an independent monitor.

An intraoperative navigation system, which incorporated port placement planning using overlay intraperitoneal images on the patient's abdominal wall, was developed by Sugimoto et al. [6]. Raw data of the preoperative patient information obtained via multiple detector computed tomography (MDCT) were used to volume rendering using OsiriX (OsiriX Fundation, Geneva, Switzerland). In order to simultaneously display the target organ and blood vessels, they injected carbon dioxide into the gastrointestinal tract and pancreatobiliary duct, and at the same time administering a rapid intravenous injection of contrast agent, then scanning, enabling the simultaneous display of the gastrointestinal tract and pancreatobiliary duct with associated blood vessels. For registration, the 3D model was set to reproduce the patient body surface, and the positional coordinates of the umbilicus, left and right nipples, and the inguinal region were fixed as physiological markers on the body surface. This registration process was non-invasive and markerlesss, and was completed within 5 min. They used the navigation system during seven surgeries, including three cholecystectomies, two gastrectomies and two colectomies. During surgery, 3D volume-rendering reconstructions of the gastrointestinal tract, blood vessels and soft tissue were projected on the patient's abdomen, and therefore unexpected organ injury could be avoided when the port was inserted. In laparoscopic biliary surgery, the displayed virtual cholangiography with surrounding vessel anatomy on the abdominal wall reduced the number of ports during surgery.

A real-time AR navigation system to be used in an open MRI operating theater was presented by Tsutsumi et al. [29]. The system was used during a laparoscopic cholecystectomy in three patients and during a laparoscopic ventral hernia repair in two patients. The operating theater was equipped with a 0.4-T open MRI, an optical tracking system and MR-compatible equipment such as a surgical bed, surgical lights, a respirator, a display monitor, and vital monitoring systems. To perform the laparoscopic interventions they used MR-incompatible surgical instruments, but out of the 5G restriction area as much as possible. For each patient, they place six to nine skin-affixed MRI-visible markers on the patient abdomen as well as the surgical ports. Then, an initial MRI scan was performed under the pneumoperitoneum, so that they can obtain the 3D model of the anatomical structures with the possible deformations caused by the pneumoperitoneum. Registration between the patient and the MRI images was performed by recording the space location of the skin-affixed markers on the patient using a handle probe registered by the optical tracker. Then, to the position of the laparoscope was also recorded, so that the virtual model was updated in real time with regard to the laparoscope's movement. The navigation frame rate was 8 frames per min. Laparoscopic cholecystectomy was successfully performed in three patients and laparoscopic ventral hernia repair in two patients. During the operations, the laparoscopic monitor clearly showed the AR models of the intraperitoneal structures, such as the common bile ducts and the urinary bladder (Figure 3), as well as the proper positions of the prosthesis.

Simpfendorfer et al. [30] developed an AR system that could fuse 3D models from transrectal US (TRUS) with a real laparoscopic video during radical prostatectomy. For registration of both image modalities (3D-2D), the system used custom-developed needles with colored heads that were inserted into the prostate using conventional laparoscopic instruments. Once the navigations aids were inserted, the 3D TRUS data was acquired. These navigations aids were segmented in the 3D model as well as in the 2D video images recorded from the laparoscope. By means of this registration the system was able to compensate the organ and/or camera movements. The virtual model was superimposed on the laparoscopic video stream defining the dissection borders for the prostate, the nerves and vessels. In order to avoid the risk of spreading tumor cells, the navigation aids were removed with the prostate inside the specimen bag. The initial test of the navigation system in an in vivo human patient was successfully performed and with no complications [30]. The setup of the navigation system took approximately 12 minutes in total, including the insertion of the navigation aids, the intraoperative US image acquisition, and the creation of the models. This AR method has been also used in a partial nephrectomy [9].

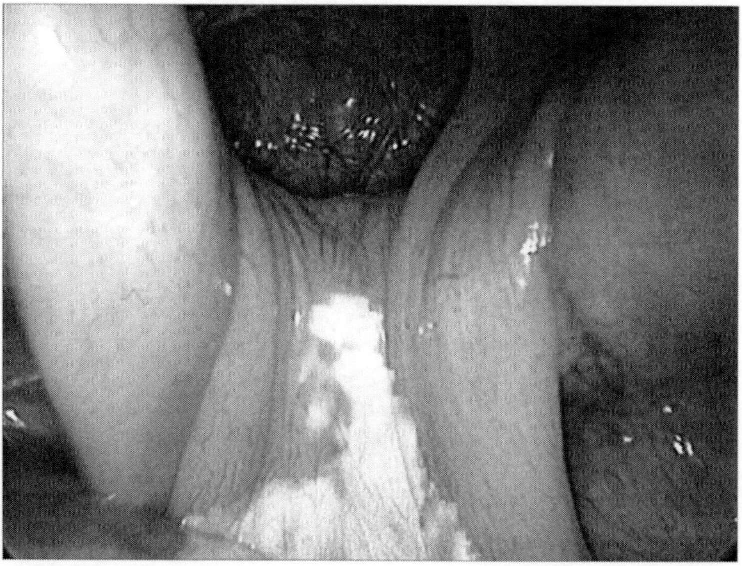

Figure 3. View of the laparoscopic monitor with overlaid polygon of the urinary bladder (Courtesy of Prof. M. Hashizume, Department of Advanced Medical Initiatives, Kyushu University, Fukuoka, Japan).

Soler et al. proposed an interactive AR method for liver resection [14]. In this case, the 3D model of the patient was adapted manually to the real model, modifying its position, scale and orientation so that visible landmarks coincided both on the 3D model and the real view of the patient. Therefore, a continuous interaction of the surgeon to update the 3D model with regard to possible intraoperative alterations was needed. Besides, this system provided resection tools for virtually resecting the 3D model during the surgical intervention. This system used CT imaging data to carry out the three steps that form the entire process: 3D patient modeling, preoperative patient visualization and virtual surgical planning and intraoperative AR assistance. For the 3D patient modeling they proposed an automatic method based on hierarchical segmentation of visible organs, from the easiest to the most complex one, using the software VR-Anat©IRCAD 2011. This interactive AR system has been applied on 40 surgical oncological procedures for liver, adrenal gland, pancreas, and parathyroid tumor resection. However, more quantitative information is needed to validate its efficiency during surgical interventions.

An AR navigation system for laparoscopic splenectomy based on preoperative MDCT was proposed by Leiri et al. [31]. For the intervention they previously segmented some important anatomical structures in the patient's 3D model such as the spleen, accessory spleen, vascular structures and pancreas, and a color-code was defined for each of them. For the registration process, five multimodality markers were placed on the patient's body, and then the MDCT scan was obtained. After scanning, the artificial markers on the patient were registered with regard to the volume image by means of an optical tracking system (Polaris, Northern Digital Inc., Ontario, Canada). After pneumoperitoneum and insertion of the scope, the registration between the spleen surface and the 3D volume was adjusted. To record the movements of the laparoscopic camera during the intervention, and therefore update the overlay images, visible infrared markers were placed on it. The overlay images were updated with about 10 fps. However, this AR navigation system does not take into account respiratory motion, pneumoperitoneum, or organ deformation. The system was used during six cases of laparoscopic splenectomy in children and all the interventions were carried out successfully. None of the cases required conversion to open surgery. During surgery, the splenic artery, splenic vein, and pancreas were fused onto laparoscopic images.

2.4. Fluorescence-Guided Surgery

Another technique for IGS is the fluorescence-guided surgery (FGS), which is an imaging technique that enables to detect anatomical structures that are fluorescently labeled during surgery. This technique allows surgeons to visualize some intraabdominal structures that are not visible with a conventional laparoscope under white light, providing an additional diagnosis tool during the intervention. FGS has the potential to improve cancer surgery outcomes, minimize the time under anesthesia and reduce health-care costs by means of its improved contrast and depth of tissue penetration compared to visible light [32]. There are different fluorescent contrast agents described in the scientific literature that can be used for near-infrared fluorescence (NIRF) imaging as a tool for photodynamic diagnostic (PDD) during MIS such as indocyanine green (ICG), fluorescein or 5-aminolevulinic acid (5-ALA) [33].

Fluorescence imaging can support the diagnosis in surgical procedures such as laparoscopic hepatectomy. This procedure has some limitations compared to open hepatectomy such as the limited possibility to visualize and palpate liver surfaces that may lead to miss some subcapsular lesions during surgery. Kudo et al. [34] used this diagnostic technique in 17 patients who underwent laparoscopic hepatectomy. To this end, a dose of 0.5 mg/kg of ICG was administered intravenously within the 2 weeks prior to surgery. ICG is a fluorescent tricarbocyanine dye that absorbs near infrared light and subsequently emits light at slightly longer wavelengths. Since ICG is retained in cancerous tissues and/or non-cancerous compressed liver parenchyma around tumors, it was used during surgery as a fluorescence source. The laparoscopic fluorescence imaging system used consisted of a commercial camera (Olympus Medical Systems, Tokyo, Japan) and a cutoff filter on the camera head. Additionally, an intraoperative ultrasonography with a flexible laparoscopic probe (BK Medical, Herlev, Den-mark, or Hitachi-Aloka Medical, Tokyo, Japan) was also used to screen the whole liver. Results reported that using fluorescence imaging they were able to identify 12 hepatocellular carcinomas of the 16 cases identified (75%) and 11 liver metastases of the 16 cases identified (69%). In a study with 6 pigs, the ICG fluorescent agent was also used to detect the ischemic areas in a laparoscopic mesenteric ischemia model [35]. They injected intravenously a dose of 0.5 mg/kg 15 min after ischemia of a small bowel loop. The ICG fluorescence signal was detected using the D-Light-P laparoscope imaging system (Karl Storz GmbH & Co. KG, Tüttlingen, Germany).

Mohsen et al. [36] reported the first use in humans of fluorescein to improve visualization of biliary topography during laparoscopic cholecystectomy. This technique took advantage of the fact that the liver excretes fluorescein and ultraviolet A (UVA) excites fluorescein causing it to emit green light. A custom-made UVA source of light was used to induce fluorescence of bile. This device had an external rod with 11 mm of diameter so that it could be inserted in a 12 mm surgical port. The technique was applied to 5 patients who had symptomatic gallstones and who underwent a laparoscopic cholecystectomy. After induction of pneumoperitoneum, fluorescein sodium at 7.5 mg/kg was injected intravenously. Then, the UVA lighting device was introduced through the epigastric port and the white light from the laparoscope was reduced. In all cases the bile ducts started to show fluorescence under UVA light within 4 to 5 minutes after fluorescein injection. During the operation, the UVA light was used in three main occasions: for an initial visualization, before clipping the cystic duct and at the end, to detect possible leakage of fluorescent bile. No leakage was reported at the end of the operation. This technique allowed better and earlier real-time visualization of biliary anatomy than conventional white light. This method could be a complementary imaging technique of intraoperative cholangiography or intraoperative US. Schols et al. [37] also obtained a successful fluorescence delineation of both the cystic duct and artery using both fluorophores intravenous ICG and CW800-CA, and a commercially available laparoscopic fluorescence imaging system (Karl Storz GmbH & Co. KG). They tested the technique during a laparoscopic cholecystectomy performed in six pigs.

The use of fluorescence imaging techniques has also applied to detection of peritoneal metastasis in human colorectal cancer [38]. In this study 5-ALA was used as a fluorescent contrast agent. In cancer cells, 5-ALA causes the increase in activity of porphobilinogen deaminase and the decrease in activity of ferrochelatase, which leads to intracellular accumulation of protoporphyrin IX (PpIX). PpIX emits red fluorescence with a blue-violet light excitation (380-430 nm). This technique was tested in twelve patients with colorectal cancer. For these interventions 5-ALA hydrochloride dissolved in 20 ml of 50% glucose solution was orally administered 3 h before surgery at a dose of 15-20 mg/kg, $\leq$1 g per patient. At the beginning of the intervention, the abdominal cavity was observed in white light image as well as fluorescence image under excitation with blue-violet light and using a long pass filter on the laparoscopic camera. Peritoneal dissemination was observed in 8 patients with conventional white light observation, which were also detected with fluorescence image. A small, flat lesion was only detected using fluorescence imaging in one patient. This imaging technique has been also used as PDD in neurosurgery and urology [39, 40].

The use of infrared fluorescence imaging as PDD may help to achieve maximal nephron preservation during partial nephrectomy, and therefore avoid possible complications associated with renal insufficiency. In a study with 77 patients who underwent a laparoscopic partial nephrectomy, orally administrated 5-ALA was used for intraoperative PDD of tumor type and resection margins [41]. As imaging systems they used the D-Light-P laparoscope (Karl Storz GmbH & Co. KG). Results showed that PDD using 5-ALA was highly sensitive detecting renal cell carcinoma in dissected tumors. This diagnostic technique was able to predict the type of the lesion with an accuracy of 94% and with a positive predictive value of 98%. In another study, 2 patients underwent a laparoscopic partial nephrectomy and 17 patients a robot-assisted partial nephrectomy using ICG for PDD [42]. Before surgery, patients received intravenous injections of ICG, which was diluted to a 2.5mg/ml solution and the total doses ranged from 5mg to 25 mg until obtaining the optimal fluorescence. The intraoperative ICG fluorescence signal was visualized using the Endoscopic SPY® Imaging System (Novadaq Inc., Missisaugua, Ontario, Canada). Final results reported that 13 patients had malignant lesions, where the tumor margin demarcation was most apparent with NIRF imaging. Specifically, malignant renal tumors were visualized as hypofluorescent compared with the surrounding normal renal parenchyma.

Recently, Hockenberry et al. [43] described a novel use of NIRF imaging without ICG or other injectable contrast agents to identify otherwise obscured intraluminal areas of interest during robotic-assisted laparoscopic (RAL) surgery marked by the white light of endoscopic instruments. They used the NIRF imaging system provided by the da Vinci® Surgical System (Intuitive Surgical, Inc., Sunnyvale, CA) by means of the FireFly® integrated system (Novadaq®; Mississauga, Ontario, CA). They applied this imaging technique in five patients during different urologic RAL interventions. Using this NIRF imaging, intraoperative ureteroscopy was used to identify the extent of a ureteral stricture in a patient undergoing RAL partial ureterectomy. Cystoscopy was used to identify bladder diverticula and tumor locations in three patients undergoing RAL partial cystectomy with or without diverticulectomy and the ureteral orifice in another patient undergoing RAL nephroureterectomy. In particular, during the RAL partial ureterectomy, by filtering light wavelengths below near-infrared and accentuating the near-infrared spectrum, the intraluminal white light of the ureteroscope appears green while the surrounding structures remain visible for the laparoscopic camera, which allowed surgeons to easily identify the ureteral stricture.

3. Robot-Assisted Interventions

Compared with traditional laparoscopic surgery, robotic-assisted interventions offer advantages such as higher range of motion, 3D visualization, and scaling of movements [44]. The first robotic-assisted surgeries on humans were conducted at the beginning of 1985 using the Programmable Universal Machine for Assembly (PUMA®) model 200 developed by Unimation Company to perform CT-guided intracranial neurological biopsies. The PUMA® 200 is an industrial servo-controlled robotic arm with six degrees of freedom (DOF) that was adapted for stereotactic surgery [45,46]. Robot-assisted surgery is becoming the gold standard for urological surgeries including prostatectomy, and it seems that gynecology is the next main focus. With the continuous advances in surgical techniques and surgical robotics, it is expected that in the future all surgical treatments can be performed by endoscopic procedures or by robot-assisted surgery. However, at the moment, a robotic surgical operation is too far to be performed entirely without human control. Surgical robots are generally used for specific surgical tasks such as supporting and improving the intracorporeal suture, holding the laparoscopic camera or taking a biopsy. Although, there are some more complex robotic platforms, as the da Vinci® Surgical System, that can be used as a support to complete the entire surgical procedure.

Despite their wide benefits there are some problems that remain to be solved in robotic surgery such as the price of surgical robots and their maintenance, the size, the lack of training for surgeons, and the few available studies that confirm the improved performance and outcomes of robotic-assisted surgical procedures.

3.1. Surgical Robots for MIS

In this section, some of the most popular robotic surgical systems for MIS, which are commercially available or in their last stages of development prior commercialization, are described.

3.1.1. Automated Endoscopic System for Optimal Positioning (AESOP®)

The earliest commercial system for robotic laparoscopic surgery which was accepted by the surgical community was the Automated Endoscopic System for Optimal Positioning (AESOP®). This system was developed by Computer Motion (Santa Barbara, CA, USA), a company that was founded with grants from National Aeronautics and Space Administration (NASA) and the National Science Foundation (NSF). The AESOP® system was able to control automatically the motion of a laparoscopic camera attached to its robotic arm. This support system allows for more precise and consistent movements of the laparoscopic camera, providing surgeons with a steadier view and filling the needs for holding the camera by a surgical staff during the entire procedure. Additionally, the AESOP® system controls the motion of the camera by means of surgeon's commands transmitted by either foot pedals or voice [47]. This system was cleared by the Food and Drug Administration (FDA) in 1994 to assist surgeons in MIS.

The AESOP® camera holder has been used during routine gynecological endoscopic surgical procedures [48]. The previous study reported that the voice-controlled AESOP® works more efficiently and faster than the hand or foot control. This device has been also used during laparoscopic radical prostatectomy [49] and laparoscopic cholecystectomy, among others minimally invasive surgical procedures.

3.1.2. ZEUS® Surgical System

After the initial success with AESOP®, Computer Motion decided to develop an entire robotic surgical system with surgical manipulators based on three AESOP® arms, the ZEUS® Surgical System. Two arms were designed to host the surgical instruments and one for the laparoscopic camera. The ZEUS® Surgical System is a master-slave system with remote manipulators controlled by means of a console. The surgeon seated at the console should wear polarized glasses to perceive the 3D image form the flat monitor. In 2001 the FDA cleared Computer Motion's ZEUS® Robotic Surgical System for use in abdominal operations [50]. This surgical system provided tremor filtering and scaling function. In 2003 Computer Motion was acquired by Intuitive Surgical, discontinuing the commercialization of both AESOP® and ZEUS® robotic systems.

This surgical platform was originally designed for minimally invasive procedures such as beating heart, coronary artery bypass grafting and mitral valve repairs [51]. ZEUS® has been used to harvest internal mammary arteries [52] and to perform in 1998 the world's first robotically-assisted minimally invasive coronary artery bypass grafting at the University Hospital Munich-Grosshadern in Germany [53]. ZEUS® is also well-known for the "Lindbergh" surgery in 2001 where a surgeon in New York, USA, performed a laparoscopic cholecystectomy in Strasbourg, France, demonstrating for the first time the feasibility of telepresence surgery [50,54].

3.1.3. The da Vinci® Surgical System

The emergence of laparoscopic surgery, combined with the interest of the US Army to operate on severely wounded soldiers directly in the battlefield or in the route to a field hospital led the NASA and the Stanford Research Institute (SRI) to focus their research programs on telesurgery [55]. This initiative was significantly supported by the Defense Advanced Research Projects Agency (DARPA). Their efforts were eventually very fruitful and the research produced a robotic endoscopic surgical system. However, limitations in telecommunication and funding prevented its implementation in the battlefield. Instead, the robotic platform was adapted for civilian and commercialized by Intuitive Surgical Incorporation (Sunnyvale, CA, USA) as the da Vinci® Surgical System [56].

The da Vinci® Surgical System was first launched in 1999. The main purpose of this robotic surgical system has been to provide a reliable, intuitive, surgical platform that brings the benefits of MIS to the patient while the surgeon is performing the procedure with similar conditions to open surgery such as higher dexterity, better ergonomic conditions and 3D visualization. Initially, the ability of this surgical platform to manipulate delicate tissues was applied to cardiac surgery. Subsequently, the benefits of this surgical robotic platform were extended to other surgical disciplines.

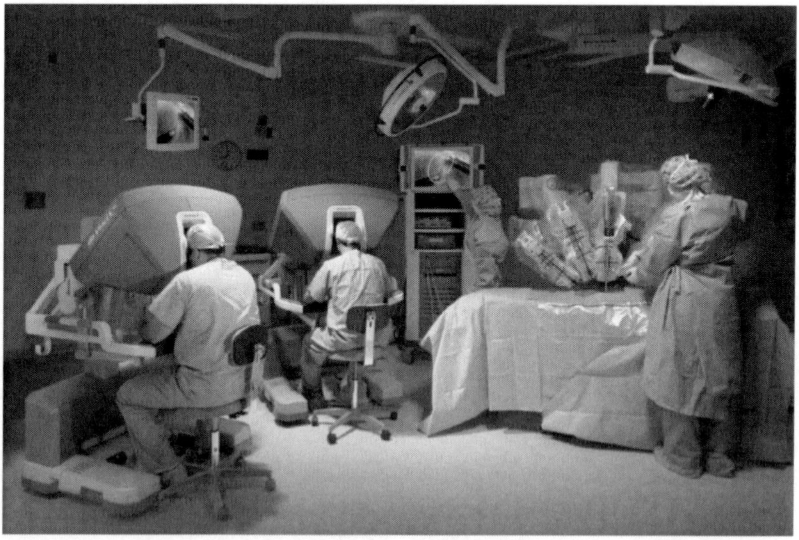

Figure 4. The da Vinci® Si System in an OR with the double console (©2014 Intuitive Surgical, Inc.).

Nowadays, the da Vinci® Surgical System is the only commercially available master-slave robotic system. At the end of 2012, there were more than 2,500 da Vinci® Surgical Systems installed in over 2,000 hospitals worldwide [56]. Therefore, at present this surgical robotic system is the most commonly used for performing minimally invasive laparoscopic surgery in humans (Figure 4).

One of the main features of this surgical system is its EndoWrist® surgical instruments (Intuitive Surgical, Inc.; Sunnyvale, CA, USA) that translate the movements of the instrument handle to the remote tip in an intuitive manner, avoiding the fulcrum effect. The end effector of these instruments mimic human hand motion by a mechanical articulation, providing surgeons with additional three DOF (seven in total) and about 90° of articulation in the wrist. These features provide surgeons with a full range of motion during the performance of minimally invasive procedures. However, not all the provided instruments are wristed such as the Harmonic® ACE and the single-site instruments. Additionally, the da Vinci® Surgical System is equipped with tremor filtering, scaling function, and alignment of the eyes and hands with the provided image of the instruments tip. The surgical image is displayed in real time through a high-quality 3D endoscope into the stereo viewer. Besides, this stereo viewer allows for additional visual information such as CT or US images.

There have been four commercial models of the da Vinci Surgical System: the da Vinci® Standard System, the da Vinci® S System (released in 2006), the da Vinci® Si Surgical System (released in 2009), and the most current version, the da Vinci® Xi System (released in 2014). The da Vinci® Standard System has been discontinued from sale and is no longer supported by Intuitive Surgical. The second version, the da Vinci® S Surgical System, was designed to facilitate surgical setup through a slimmer arm design and the addition of a fourth robotic arm. The da Vinci® Si version was equipped with a 3D full high-definition vision system, a second console for training, the availability to perform single-site surgery, and the integration of laser technology to allow for fluorescent imaging [56]. One of the most remarkable advances of the latest version, the da Vinci® Xi Surgical System, is that it allows for multi-quadrant surgery that can be performed without repositioning the system. Additionally, this version provides smaller and thinner arms as well as the ability to attach the endoscope to any arm. At the moment, Intuitive Surgical remains the market leader for robotic MIS by holding the license of more than 1,000 patents that cover the fundamental aspects of the da Vinci® Surgical System's technology such as the surgical console, the vision system and the wristed instruments. This hampers the development of new robotic surgical systems.

This surgical platform has been successfully used in a wide range of abdominal [57] and thoracic procedures [58]. In addition, it has been applied to other emerging procedures such as single-site surgery [59, 60] and Natural Orifice Transluminal Endoscopic Surgery (NOTES) [61,62] in an attempt to further reduce the invasiveness of surgery. Although this is a system for telesurgery and all robotic arms are controlled remotely from the surgical console, its installation, removal, and exchange of the camera as well as the instruments should be performed by a bedside assistant. Besides, for some interventions installation of the system is time-consuming considering that for some procedures time is a critical issue. Although the latest version, the da Vinci® Xi System, seems to have improved this limitation.

3.1.4. Amadeus® Surgical System

Similar to the da Vinci® Surgical System, another project that is currently under development is the Amadeus® system (Titan Medical Inc., Toronto, Canada), which is a 4-armed robotic surgical platform for MIS with snakelike multiarticulating arms for improved maneuverability and obstacle avoidance [63]. As the da Vinci® Surgical System this surgical platform consists of a master-salve robotic system with a workstation that allows surgeon to control remotely the robotic surgical instruments. This workstation also provides surgeon with 3D endoscopic view of the surgical field and a set of instruments for single-site surgery. In addition, this system includes force feedback for detection of tissue-level forces, which allows surgeons to feel how hard they are pulling on tissues, sutures, or other structures, minimizing tissue damage. Currently, the company has put the Amadeus system on the back burner to focus their efforts on developing and commercializing a new robotic platform for Single-Site Surgery, the Titan's Single Port Orifice Robotic Technology (SPORT™) surgical system.

3.2. Robotic Surgery in MIS

The introduction of laparoscopic surgery came with some technical limitations including mirroring of instrument movements, limited articulation, two-dimensional (2D) visualization and poor ergonomics, which may lead to some surgical complications [64]. These technical limitations of laparoscopic surgery significantly influenced the development of robotic surgical systems as a means to improve the control of laparoscopic instruments, providing wider maneuverability in complex procedures, and improve visualization of the surgical field. Some advantages of robotic surgical systems include 3D vision, increased precision and dexterity, and ergonomic conditions for the surgeon that may lead to less muscle fatigue. However, in order to ensure the success of a robotic procedure, a variety of factors must be taken into account such as the surgical system to be used, the appropriate selection of surgical equipment as well as patient and procedural considerations.

3.2.1. Robotic-assisted Urological Surgery

Robotic was first introduced in urological surgery in 1991 to conduct a transurethral resection of the prostate using the robotic system Probot® (Imperial College, London, UK), a resection device with seven DOF. For this procedure, the surgical robot was used to insert into the patient a cutting device for removing the prostatic tissue. This system possesses a transurethral ultrasonographic probe at its tip to measure the gland at the beginning of the procedure, providing an intraabdominal model of the prostate in which the surgeon can define the area to be removed. Then, the robotic system computes the trajectories of resection for the surgical tool and follows them during the intervention [65].

There are a substantial number of studies on performing complex urological procedures with robotic assistance in humans that has documented their safety, efficacy, and feasibility [66]. These studies have applied robotic-assisted surgery to several urological domains such as localized prostate cancer (radical prostatectomy), bladder cancer (radical cystectomy and urinary diversion for muscle-invasive bladder cancer), kidney surgery (nephrectomy, donor nephrectomy, partial nephrectomy), pyelo-ureteric junction obstruction (pyeloplasty), and adrenal surgery [67].

The first successful laparoscopic radical prostatectomy was performed by Schuessler in 1991 [68]. However, due to its technical difficulty, this operation was not widely carried out until the da Vinci® surgical system appeared. The miniature tools with EndoWrist® technology offer a potential advantage over standard laparoscopic instruments in the accuracy of movements and suturing along with high-magnification 3D view. This ensures preservation of the lateral prostatic fascia, which may result in better erectile function postoperatively as compared to conventional open surgery [69,70]. RAL radical prostatectomy seems to reduce the blood loss, risk of intraoperative transfusion, and anastomotic strictures in comparison with retropubic radical prostatectomy [71]. Consequently, this new technology has spread rapidly, and in 2009 about 85 % of all radical prostatectomies in the USA were performed by assistance of the da Vinci® surgical system [67,72].

In the case of partial nephrectomy, although open approach remains the reference standard for the treatment of small renal tumors, laparoscopic partial nephrectomy is constantly evolving. However, this is a challenging approach due to its steep learning curve and technical requirements. To cope with some of these limitations, robotic technology has recently been applied to laparoscopic partial nephrectomy with the goal of providing a safe and effective alternative to laparoscopic partial nephrectomy [73]. The first robot-assisted partial nephrectomy was described by Gettman et al. [74] in 2004. Some studies suggested that RAL partial nephrectomy offers equivalent oncological control to open and laparoscopic partial nephrectomy while reporting shorter hospital stay, less intraoperative blood loss, shorter operating room time and shorter warm ischemia time [73,75,76].

3.2.2. Robotic-assisted Cardiac Surgery

The application of laparoscopic techniques to cardiac surgery entails some difficulties such as the lack of dexterity using the conventional laparoscopic instrumentation that is required for delicate cardiac surgical procedures and the loss of depth perception due to the 2D vision. The application of robotic technology has overcome some of these limitations, providing new approaches to minimally invasive cardiac surgery.

In 1998 Stephenson et al. [77] reported the first robot-assisted totally endoscopic coronary anastomosis on twenty-five isolated porcine hearts placed inside a thoracic trainer, using an arterial conduit to the left anterior descending artery. The procedure was performed endoscopically using the ZEUS® Surgical System [77]. All the 25 surgeries were successfully completed and showed good probe patency. The lack of tremor and motion scaling allowed for the precise movements required to complete the endoscopic microvascular anastomosis. Loulmet et al. applied the first robotic totally endoscopic coronary artery bypass grafting in humans in 1998 [78]. This intervention was performed in 4 male patients with the indication of grafting the left internal thoracic artery to the left anterior descending coronary artery. The da Vinci® Surgical System was used to perform the surgery and the Heartport® system (Heartport, Inc, Redwood City, USA) was used for arresting the heart during the anastomosis. Carpentier et al. [79] performed the first robotic mitral valve repair using an early prototype of the da Vinci® Surgical System in 1998.

The FDA approved the da Vinci® Surgical System for mitral valve surgery in 2002 and in 2004 for use in coronary anastomosis during cardiac revascularization. Some of the most common applications of robot-assisted cardiac surgery are the mitral valve repair [80] and endoscopic coronary artery bypass grafting [81,82]. Over 1,700 robotic cardiac operations per year are currently performing in the USA and the numbers are increasing each year [83].

The CardioARM® is one of the latest surgical robots that have being introduced is in the field of cardiac surgery. CardioArm® was developed at Carnegie Mellon University (Pittsburgh, USA). This system consists of a slim snakelike manipulator designed to perform minimally invasive epicardial interventions through a subxiphoid approach. The CardioARM® was developed in an effort to provide dedicated intrapericardial therapeutic delivery with single port access. One of the main advantages of this design is the ability to preserve its previous configuration and shape in intraabdominal space during navigation or to become completely flexible if necessary [84].

3.2.3. Robotic-assisted Thoracic Surgery

The application of MIS to thoracic surgery has been slow mainly due to some difficulties that entail this type of surgery such as the limited thoracic space, the ribs restrictions, the heartbeat and the breathing [85]. The initial application of video-assisted thoracic surgery was only as a diagnostic tool. The development of specific thoracoscopic instruments led to more complex procedures such as pulmonary lobectomy. Apart from its technical demand, thoracoscopic surgery has a steep learning curve because of the unergornomic position and two-dimensional view. In this sense, advances in robotic surgery have tried to solve some of these limitations.

Several cases have been reported in which robotic-assisted thoracoscopic surgery has been performed for the early-stages of lung cancer [86,87]. Jang HJ et al. [88] compared the results of forty cases of robot-assisted lobectomy (RAL) with forty cases of video-assisted thoracic surgery lobectomy (VAL) for lung cancer. Results showed no conversions to open thoracotomy in RAL against 2% for the VAL group. The operative time for both surgical techniques was similar, but the rate of postoperative complications in the RAL group (n = 4) was significantly lower than that of the VAL group (n = 13). Additionally, postoperative stay was significantly shorter for the RAL (6 vs 9 days). Park et al. [89] reported that the cost in the USA of video-assisted or robotic-assisted thoracic surgery for lung cancer was lower than open thoracotomy due to the longer hospital stay than this later required.

The mediastinum, especially the upper part, is a delicate and difficult anatomical area to be reached through thoracoscopy mainly because this anatomical area has large and fragile vessels and nerves. Thoracoscopic surgery has some limitations that make those maneuvers more difficult such as the 2D view of the surgical field and the lack of DOF of the surgical instruments that limit the maneuverability. The thoracoscopic thymectomy is considered a technically challenging operation that requires a long learning curve [90]. The introduction of robotic surgical system has dealt with some of the aforementioned problems, mainly the increasing in maneuverability compared to conventional thoracoscopy [85]. However, the lack of tactile feedback of most of the current robotic systems may increase the risk to damage the tumor tissue, increasing the possibility of tumor seeding.

3.2.4. Robotic-assisted Gynecological Surgery

Since its approval for use in gynecologic surgery by the FDA in 2005, the da Vinci® Surgical System has been widely adopted by hospitals and gynecologic surgeons [91]. At the moment, it is the only commercially available robotic surgical platform for gynecologic surgery in the US. The application of robotic technology has had a strong impact in abdominal and pelvic surgery. One of the most influential results is a decrease in the number of procedures performed by laparotomy, even in the case of obesity, which leads to a reduction in blood loss, shorter hospitalization, and shorter recovery to normal activities [92,93]. Magrina et al. [92] reported a 3% of conversion rate with robotic surgery for endometrial cancer in comparison to 10% for laparoscopic patients. Robotic-assisted surgery has been extensively applied in gynecological surgery in benign gynecology as well as gynecologic oncology. Robotic-assisted surgery allows gynecologists to perform minimally invasive hysterectomies [94], myomectomies [95], and lymph node biopsies [96] without the need for large abdominal incisions.

3.3. Robotic Single-Site Surgery

Since the introduction of laparoscopy, MIS has experienced great advances and innovation, in the pursuit of the final objective to eliminate or keep invisible all scars after surgery. In this sense, laparoendoscopic single-site surgery (LESS) is now consolidated as a real alternative to conventional laparoscopic surgery, with numerous studies sustaining its feasibility and therapeutic safety [97-99]. In this new approach, articulated or prebent instruments are introduced into the abdominal cavity through specific multichannel ports or conventional low profile laparoscopic trocars, placed in close proximity through one single incision. If the surgical procedure is performed with an additional transperitoneal port, it is referred to as hybrid LESS. This way, and still lacking scientific proof, single incision offers various theoretical or potential advantages, such as better cosmetic results, lower incidence of incisional pain, and faster recovery. This surgical technique particularly contributes to excellent cosmesis results mainly because of the surgical scars are often undetectable, especially when the surgical entrance is through the umbilicus.

Apart from its benefits, LESS surgery presents some specific difficulties, which include the reduction in freedom of movement, inline vision with loss of triangulation [100], and closer proximity of instruments, leading to external and intraabdominal clashing and crossing [101], and the deficient ergonomy for the operating surgeon [102]. Clashing of instruments could be partially avoided by using prebent, articulated or instruments of different lengths. Additionally, when using flexible instruments, the size and weight of tissue that can be held are limited owing to the insufficient force transmitted through the instruments.

In an attempt to overcome these problems, new specifically designed instruments and devices are being developed. In this regard, robotic systems for LESS may improve the ability to maneuver within the abdominal cavity due to the possibility of use articulated robotic instruments and with higher number of DOF. This has led to a new kind of surgery, robotic LESS or R-LESS. R-LESS promises to overcome the limitations of laparoscopic single-site surgery by eliminating instrument clashing and reproducing conventional triangulation in a single incision environment. However, further developments are needed in order to optimize the current robotics systems to single-site surgery.

3.3.1. Da Vinci® Surgical System

The first application of single-site robotics in gynecology was reported by Escobar et al. using standard EndoWrist® instruments directed through a GelPort® (Applied Medical; Rancho Santa Margarita, USA) through the umbilicus [103]. Also Kaouk et al. reported the first clinical cases in humans of robotic single-site surgery for radical prostatectomy, radical nephrectomy, and dismembered pyeloplasty using the da Vinci® S Surgical System [104]. In July 2009, White et al. [105] mentioned the first clinical cases of R-LESS uretral reimplant and sacral colpopexy. The first application of R-LESS in digestive surgery was reported by Ostrowitz et al. [106]. Romanelli et al. [107] mentioned the first R-LESS cholecystectomy and Allemann et al. [108] reported the performance of a Nissen fundoplication on 18 pigs either with R-LESS or LESS.

In 2009, Intuitive Surgical Inc. released the third generation of da Vinci® Surgical System, the da Vinci® Si System, which included a wide range of specialized instruments for single-site surgery, a surgical simulator and near-infrared imaging capabilities [109]. The da Vinci® Single-Site Instrumentation kit contains material that has been specifically designed to enable robotic surgery through a single incision of 2-2.5 cm. These surgical instruments are inserted thorough curved trocars, and therefore avoiding collisions between the robotic arms. Additionally, the robotic system can switch the instruments in the right and left side on the control panel, which allows the surgeon to manipulate the instruments on the console as they were not crossed [44]. These new instruments for LESS have been tested for cholecystecmy [59], pyeloplasty [60] and nephrectomies procedures [109], amount others.

However, the flexible instruments for R-LESS provided by Intuitive Surgical are not wristed, and therefore the surgical performance is as if straight-stick conventional laparoscopy instruments were using. In addition, the flexible instrument shafts, necessary for instrument delivery through curved cannulas, limit the tolerance for load of the instruments, causing the shaft could be bent when it has excessive load.

3.3.2. Single-Port Laparoscopy Bimanual Robot (SPRINT®)

The SPRINT® is a master-slave teleoperated robotic platform developed for bimanual interventions by means of single access port. This system consists of two robotic arms with a maximum diameter of 18 mm and a stereoscopic camera (Karl Storz GmbH & Co. KG). This device mounts two graspers that differ in shape and size, which are controlled using a wire-driven mechanism (Figure 5). Each grasper can applied up to 5 N of force. Each robotic arm has embedded the motors and gear boxes, which provide them six DOF. The surgeon's console consists of two manipulators for each of the robotic arms, one pedal and a 3D Full-HD vision system with polarized glasses. Two Phantom Omni haptic devices (Sensable Technologies Inc., Woburn, USA) are used as manipulator, thus enabling to control all six DOF of each robotic arm. This robotic system is still in the prototype phase and still presents some mechanical constraints [110].

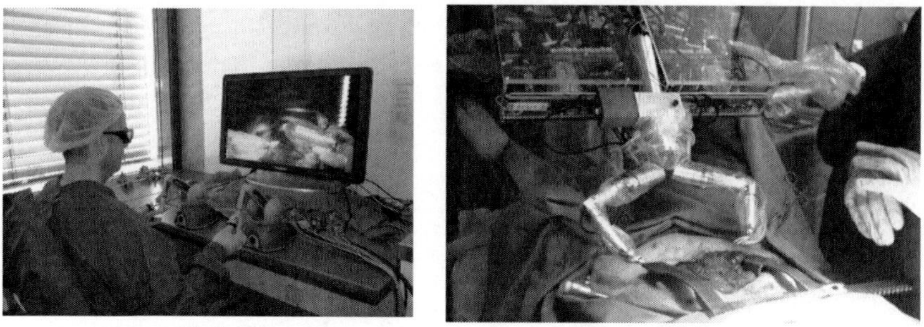

(a) (b)

Figure 5. SPRINT® robot for single-site surgery. (a) Surgeon console with the manipulators and the 3D monitor. (b) SPINT® robot setup in the OR (Images from [111]. Reprinted with permission).

The initial tests of this surgical system have been carried out on an in vivo animal model. A midline laparotomy of (approximately 10 cm) was performed and the abdominal cavity was exposed by means of a fixed retractor. The robotic system was fixed to the OR table and suspended over the incision made in the abdomen of the patient. A surgeon controlled remotely both arms of the robotic system during the performance of a small-bowel enteroenterostomy [111].

3.3.3. Plate- Spring Mechanism-Based Laparoscopic Surgery Robot (PLAS®)

The PLAS® prototype consists of two flexible arms assembled in a Y-shaped design [112]. Unlike the traditional wire- or link-driven mechanisms used to move the instrument arms [111], this device uses a novel plate-spring mechanism, which provides more than 14 N force transmission. This high force transmission allows for performing a wide range of surgical procedures through single port access. In contrast to the bulkiness of gearboxes and the weaknesses of wired systems, plate springs can deal with these limitations. The movements of both arms could achieve a total of 12 DOF. This feature could be one of the most competitive with regard to the other similar robotic systems, allowing the device to reach a wide workspace inside the abdominal cavity. This system has been only experimentally tested on in vivo animal models. During these experiments, a surgeon performed a liver dissection using PLAS®, determining that it has sufficient force transmission capability to handle the organs during surgery [112].

Nevertheless, the current version of PLAS® does not have an additional supporting structure to hold the endoscope and tool change is not possible.

Therefore, several ports and forceps might be required to perform an entire procedure. In addition, this device does not provide haptic feedback from the end effectors to the user's manipulators.

3.4. Robotic Natural Orifice Transluminal Endoscopic Surgery

The concept of natural orifice transluminal endoscopic surgery, most commonly known as NOTES, constitutes a new surgical approach that combines aspects of flexible endoscopy and laparoscopy, where the ultimate goal is to ensure the absence of scars in the skin of the patient. NOTES can be performed as a hybrid procedure, in case surgeon requires laparoscopic assistance or as a pure procedure, if no accessory trocar through the patient's abdominal wall is needed.

This type of surgical approach avoids the need to make any abdominal incisions, which may correlate with fewer wound infections and a faster recovery and return to daily life. Available literature confirms the feasibility and security in the short term of a variety of transluminal procedures, including cholecystectomy, appendectomy, tubal ligation, gastrojejunostomy, nephrectomy, pancreatectomy and splenectomy [113-115]. The body's orifices are considered natural routes, and reported entrances to the abdominal cavity include transgastric, transcolonic, transvaginal and transvesical. Once the transluminal procedures are completed, the endoscope is withdrawn through the natural orifice and the incision is closed by using clips or endoscopic suturing devices.

Some of the limitations of this technique include inefficient tissue traction, inadequate triangulation of instruments, and existing risk of abdominal infections due to an incorrect disinfection or visceral closing. In NOTES, to perform the surgical procedures, surgeons have to manipulate endoscopic forceps through the flexible endoscopic channel, which in some cases it does not provide the degree of maneuverability required to perform the procedure without complications. Additionally, current endoscopes and instruments remain inadequate to perform complex surgeries by NOTES approach. NOTES itself requires the acquisition of new equipment and surgical skills for deployment in the surgery, which demands for the development of specific training programs.

To overcome the aforementioned limitations, the use of robotic technology could provide a potential solution to increase the dexterity in manipulating the endoscopic forceps in a narrow visual field and a small cavity. This leads to the concept of robotic natural orifice transluminal surgery (R-NOTES).

3.4.1. Da Vinci® Surgical System

The use of the da Vinci® Surgical System for robotic-assisted NOTES has been reported in animal and cadaveric models, but not in the case of human patients. The initial experience with robotic natural orifice transluminal surgery (R-NOTES) using the da Vinci® Surgical System was reported by Haber et al. [116] for reconstructive urology. In this study, they performed 10 robotic-assisted hybrid transvaginal NOTES pyeloplasties, 10 radical and 10 partial nephrectomies in 10 in vivo porcine models. For performing these procedures, the robotic laparoscope and the first robotic arm were placed through a single umbilical incision by means of a single-port multicannula, and the second robotic arm was placed through the vagina. All the procedures were performed successfully without any open conversion or additional laparoscopic port. In a study with 3 female cadavers, two different approaches for retroperitoneal transvaginal R-NOTES nephrectomy were reported using the da Vinci® Si System in a 3-arm configuration [61]. In the first approach, the peritoneal cavity was accessed in the lithotomy position and in the prone jackknife position during the second approach. Access to the peritoneal cavity was obtained by means of a single-port device inserted through the vagina. The results showed that the first approach could not be successfully performed due to collision of the robotic arms against the legs and limited bowel retraction. During the second approach, in one of the subjects there was a rectal injury during the access and the procedures could not be completed because they could not reach the kidney with the robotic instruments due to the height of the subject. Using also a cadaveric model, Eyraud et al. [62] completed successfully a transrectal hybrid R-NOTES nephrectomy and adrenalectomy.

Demura et al. [117] analyzed the feasibility of using the da Vinci® Surgical System for a transrectal small intestinal anastomosis and closure of the rectal anterior wall incision in a porcine ex vivo model. A Tuebingen MIC trainer (Richard Wolf GmbH, Knittlingen, Germany) was used as surgical setting, in which the ex vivo small vowel segments were place. Surgical performance using the R-NOTES approach was compared with traditional transabdominal robot-assisted surgical approach as well as using transanal endoscopic microsurgery instruments (TEM NOTES). For the R-NOTES procedure, two 8-mm robotic arms were inserted through the anterior rectal wall orifice of the box trainer and placed horizontally, and a 12-mm camera was inserted through the same orifice and placed above the two arms. The number of experiments with each approach was 12. Results showed that the mean burst pressures in the transrectal R-NOTES group and the transabdominal robotic group were significantly higher than in the TEM NOTES group. Besides, the surgical time was shorter in the R-NOTES group than in the TEM NOTES group, but longer than the transabdominal robotic group.

Although the use of the da Vinci® Surgical System provides several benefits for the surgeon such as the increase dexterity, multiple DOF and 3D vision, using this robotic system for NOTES is still technically challenging. For this reason, further refinements of this technique as well as development of new surgical instruments and devices should be done. On the other hand, novel surgical devices and prototypes focus on providing new alternatives for R-NOTES are described below.

3.4.2. Endoscopic Surgical Robot for Tele-NOTES

In 2009 Suzuki et al. [118] reported the first telesurgery experiment by performing a NOTES procedure (Tele-NOTES). In this experiment they used an endoscopic surgical robot inserted through the esophagus to perform surgeries in the upper gastric tubes and the abdominal cavity through the stomach wall. Therefore, this surgical robot was able to perform intraabdominal surgeries without any external incision on the patient. The robotic system consisted of one central camera and two robotic arms, which were controlled by means of a wire-driven mechanism. The surgeon controlled the system from a surgical console, which consisted of two haptic devices (PHANTOM Omni, SensAble Technologies Inc., MA, USA) for the manipulation of forceps (Figure 6). The robot could perform grasping, incising and clipping of soft tissue using the cooperative action of left and right robotic arms.

The system has been previously used for endoscopic mucosal resection in stomach, and NOTES procedures on liver, gall bladder, small intestine and oviduct in animal models [118]. For the Tele-NOTES experiment they performed a lymph node dissection between Japan and Thailand (distance of about 3,750 km) using a human soft cadaver. The robotic system was controlled by the cooperative direction of a surgeon and an endoscopist. The surgeon was placed on the surgical console in Japan, who was in charge of manipulating the robotics arms. The endoscopist was on the patient side in Thailand controlling the endoscope.

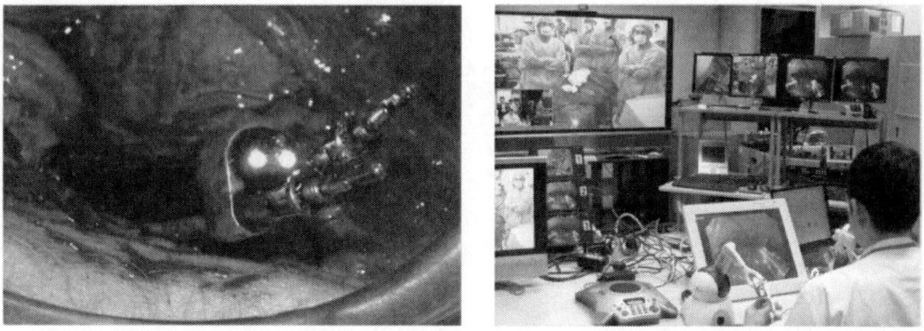

Figure 6. Endoscopic surgical robot for Tele-NOTES. (a) Surgical robot inside the abdominal cavity. (b) Remote operation unit to control the robotic arms (Courtesy of Prof. M. Hashizume, Department of Advanced Medical Initiatives, Kyushu University, Fukuoka, Japan).

3.4.3. EndoSAMURAI®

The EndoSAMURAI® (Olympus Corp., Tokyo, Japan) is a prototype platform consisting mainly of an endoscope and a control console. This endoscopic platform has two independent end effectors with five DOF, a third conventional working channel, and an ergonomic user interface [119]. The main advantage is that the console has similar actuators used in conventional laparoscopic surgery, thereby adapting to the use of the system is usually less complex and more intuitive for a laparoscopist. The two articulating working arms can be moved out of the original diameter of the scope and therefore provide more triangulation. However, this may reduce the maneuverability in tight spaces lumen such as in the oesophagus or small bowel. The system has some similar functions to a traditional endoscope such as the light source and insufflation of gas, but also standard functions for suction and the possibility of rinsing the endoscopic lens. Exchangeable instruments via the working channels of the scope allow for a variety of working functions including grasping, retracting, tissue cutting, coagulation, hemostasis, and suturing with a needle holder. In general, the system is operated by two individuals: the main surgeon placed at the workstation and the camera assistant who guides the endoscope within the abdominal cavity [120].

This device has been compared in a benchtop simulation with a conventional dual-channel endoscope during the performance of bimanual coordination tasks such as suturing and knot-tying [119]. Results showed better results for the novel device in time and accuracy. Recently, the EndoSAMURAI® has been tested in an experimental in vivo porcine model by performing a transgastric small bowel segmental resection with acceptable quality and within a reasonable time (110 min) [120].

3.4.4. Master and Slave Transluminal Endoscopic Robot (MASTER®)

Another robotic prototype for NOTES that is used with a conventional endoscope is the MASTER® (Nan Yang Technological University, Singapore). This consists of two small cable-driven flexible arms with nine DOF located at the tip of the endoscope. These cables have the enough size to be inserted through the channels of a conventional flexible endoscope with double channels. Moreover, this robotic platform provides a console for the manipulation of the surgical tools in a more intuitive manner. This console is adapted to the surgeon's needs allowing for a more ergonomic position during the intervention. The master controller is attached to the wrist and fingers of the operator and connected to the manipulator by electrical and wire cables [121]. The robotic arms allow for tissue manipulation, triangulation, off-axis forces and monopolar cautery. This system also requires an endoscopist as well as a robotic operator to perform a surgical intervention. However, there are some limitations that should be improved in future versions such as automation of camera control and an easier exchange of instrument.

This device has already been tested in ex vivo and in vivo animal models for endoscopic submucosal dissection. The novel device has been shown to have faster learning curve than using conventional endoscopic equipment to complete the procedure [121]. Recently, Phee et al. [122] performed the same procedure in 5 human patients with early-stage gastric neoplasia, limited to the mucosa. After markings and circumferential mucosal incision, all submucosal dissections were performed using the MASTER® system. All surgeries were successfully performed with no residual or recurrent tumors. Additionally, the MASTER® system has been used to perform wedge hepatic resection through the transgastric route on two female pigs. Results showed that the procedure using the novel device was accomplished successfully in both patients without the need for assistance using laparoscopic instruments [123].

3.4.5. Miniature Robot for NOTES

The robotic systems for NOTES based on the endoscope that use cable-driven arms are prone to generate friction during wire actuation inside the endoscopic channels. This may cause significant amount of hysteresis and ineffective force transmission, thus resulting in lack of instrument responsiveness and accuracy [124]. An alternative to this problem is to use systems that do not require cable-driven mechanism as the miniature robot for

NOTES developed at the University of Nebraska-Lincoln (Lincoln, USA) [125]. This device, with tubular shape, consists of two arms connected to a central body by a rotational joint. This miniature robot has two remotely controlled actuators with six DOF, stereovision and ultra bright LED lighting. Both cautery and forceps are the end-effectors provided by this device. The actuators are remotely controlled by the surgeon using an external console, which consists of two joysticks for controlling the robotic arms and a TFT color LCD monitor located between the two joysticks to display the video from the endoscopic camera.

In order to be introduced into the peritoneal cavity through the esophagus by means of a standard therapeutic endoscope, this system acquires initially a linear configuration. Once the system is inside the abdominal cavity it is restructured again into three parts using an external magnetic handle that interacts with magnets housed in the robot body. The exterior magnet handle can be moved along the outer surface of the abdomen for repositioning the robot throughout the procedure. This robotic system has been tested for an abdominal exploration, a bowel manipulation, and a cholecystectomy in three ex vivo porcine models [125]. Results of this study reported that the robot has the sufficient flexibility for transgastric insertion while providing a stable platform for tissue manipulation and visualization of the surgical field. Besides, the robotic arms were able to provide the sufficient force for tissue retraction and dissection during the procedures. However, this system experienced some problems during the execution of some of these surgical procedures. In one case, the robotic device did not have the enough magnetic coupling for attaching the robot to the interior abdominal wall and, in another procedure, there was a mechanical failure in one of its shoulder joints.

3.5. Image-guided Robotic Surgery

The principal disadvantage of the conventional endoscopic technique is that it is difficult to maintain precise control of the endoscopic instruments because of limited range of movements of the surgical instruments, heartbeat, breathing movements, instable visualization of the operative field, and haptic input. These limitations make difficult to perform some procedures that need for high precise movements such as tumor resection or cardiac surgery. In this sense, robotic technology along with image-guided techniques is a feasible solution to cope with these surgical requirements. Needles, slender probes or other instruments can be inserted into the body using real-time feedback of different imaging modalities, such as CT, MRI, US and fluoroscopy [27]. In this sense, we will focus our attention on robotic systems that are placed in imaging devices using them during the curse of the intervention.

3.5.1. Tumor Therapy

One of the most popular robotic platform for tumor ablation is the CyberKnife® system (Accuray, Inc., Sunnyvale, USA), which was the first image-guided robotic system for noninvasive radiation procedures. This robotic system was developed in 1987 as an interventional radiological robot and received the FDA approval in 2001. It consists of a large robotic arm that can quickly and accurately deliver targeted radiation with converged beams from multiple angles, reducing radiation exposure to surrounding tissue [126]. Before the intervention, a CT scan of the patient is imported into the treatment planning system. Then, the robotic manipulator automatically follows a fixed preplanned path to target the lesion, but this path can be modified automatically along the treatment on the basis of possible patient displacement. Because the patient is in continuous motion and the interior of the human body is an unstable scenario, CyberKnife® updates its spatial registration of the patient prior to each dose using an X-ray imaging system and a respiratory tracking system to track and anticipate respiratory motion [127,128]. The X-ray images are used during the treatment to compute the changes in position of the patient using the CT images as baseline, and therefore making continuous adjustments for movement. This image-guided robotic system has been used for radiotherapy of brain tumors, lesions of the spine, lung, pancreas, liver, and prostate [126].

In 2012 The Indian Perfint Healthcare Corporation (Chennai, India) released the MAXIO® system, which is an integrated planning, navigation and robotic targeting system for CT-guided tumor ablation. The use of this platform can be divided into four phases: Image registration, planning, treatment and verification. Once the CT images have been obtained, the next step is the image segmentation using a semi-automatic segmentation method. After the image segmentation has been performed and the tumor has been localized, surgeons can plan the interventional procedure in 3D by selecting the target and entry point. In this phase, the clinician can analyze the best approach to reach the tumor. Once the planning is done, clinicians can uses the MAXIO®'s robotic targeting system to support them to reach the tumor safely and as planned, and then proceed to deliver the thermal or other energy beams to blast the tumor. Finally, the visualization tools help clinicians to verify and extend the procedure if needed. The robotic platform has been tested using abdominal phantoms [129]. Initial experiences with the system reported that it improves the accuracy of needle placement, reduce number of needle passes, and significantly reduce the total radiation dose to the patients [130].

3.5.2. Cardiac Surgery

Robots have been also applied to support the intravascular procedures. In this sense, Hansen Medical (Mountain View, CA, USA) developed the Sensei® robotic catheter, which is a master-slave system that allows surgeon to control remotely a fluoroscopically guided catheter. This system prevents the exposure to radiation by the cardiologist. Sensei® received the FDA clearance in 2007. This robotic system has a workstation with an intuitive interface that translates the surgeon's hands movements to a robotically steered guided catheter using advanced robotic technology (Artisan® Control Catheter). The combination of outer and inner guide motion allows the catheter to easily acquire any curved shape. The workstation provides the fluoroscopic view of the catheter as well as the 3D model of it. Sensei® is compatible with multiple imaging systems including fluoroscopy as well as 3D mapping systems. This system also provides force feedback thanks to a force sensor at the tip of the catheter that registers the information regarding the contact between the catheter and the tissue [131]. These features allow surgeons to navigate flexible catheters with greater stability and control during complex cardiac arrhythmia procedures. This system has been used extensively for catheter ablation of atrial fibrilation [132,133]. Studies reported that the use of this system reduces fluoroscopy times in catheter ablation of atrial fibrilation, resulting in reduced X-ray exposure for patients and other surgical staff in the OR [133,134].

Another feasible option for remote catheter navigation and ablation is the use of remote magnetic navigation technology. This technology is used by the Niobe® Navigation System (Stereotaxis, St. Louis, MO, USA), which was designed for cardiac interventions. This system consists of two permanent magnets positioned at either side of the fluoroscopy table creating a spherical uniform magnetic field, which can apply a low-intensity magnetic field to the patient. The system uses a special catheter containing small magnetic implants, which are aligned with regard to the magnetic field applied. The workstation of this robotic platform is able to integrate real-time imaging data to produce 3D magnetic vectors. This allows the cardiologist to guide the tip of the catheter though the major vessels and heart of the patient by changing the orientation of the magnetic field. The Niobe® system has been proven safe and effective in the treatment of different types of supraventricular and ventricular arrhythmias [135-137].

3.5.3. MRI-compatible Robots

In 2008 Hashizume et al. [138] presented a MR image-guided surgical robotic system for MIS. The system consists of MR image guidance, an MRI-compatible operating table, an MRI-compatible master-slave surgical manipulator, and an open-bone MRI scanner (Figure 7). The master-slave robotic system is made of MRI-compatible material, and enables each manipulator to be attached to any position on the guide rail of the operating table. The manipulator system has four arms: one holds the endoscope while the other three arms hold the robotic forceps or other surgical instruments such as ablation needle, grasper, scissors or needle holder. All of them are MRI-compatible. The surgeon controls remotely the slave manipulators by means of a console, which also provides the image-guidance system and the endoscopic view. The image-guidance system allows surgeon to make a preoperative plan using the 3D anatomical images and see in real time the navigation images during the intervention in order to reach easily the target.

They performed in vivo experiments with MR image-guided laparoscopic radiofrequency ablation for liver tumors on three pigs, using mimic tumors made of agarose gel and with a diameter of approximately 2cm. In order to plan the puncture path, the surgeon segmented the target and defined the entry point on the abdominal wall using the MRI data on the preoperative planning system. Then, during the intervention the tumor was punctured using the MR image-guided surgical robotic system. The surgeon succeeded in puncturing safely all liver targets on each subject while maintaining the operative field with the robotic forceps [138].

Another MRI-compatible system for MIS is the MrBot® (Johns Hopkins Bayview Medical Center, Baltimore, USA). This is a fully-actuated robot for image-guided access of the prostate gland. The robot was customized for transperineal needle insertion and designed to be MRI-compatible. To achieve it the robot was made of nonmagnetic and dielectric materials such as plastics, ceramics, and rubbers and it is electricity free. The robot implements a pneumatic actuator to avoid electricity use. The robotic system consists of a controller unit located outside the imager's room, which has all the electric components, and the robot. The robot's end-effector has six DOF to be placed and oriented. This end-effector has an additional DOF to set the depth of needle insertion and three DOFs to manipulate a titanium needle. This robotic system has been designed to accommodate various needle drivers for different percutaneous interventions such as biopsy, thermal ablations, or brachytherapy. However, to date only the needle driver for the transperineal seed brachytherapy has been implemented. The tip of the robot has a MRI-visible set of markers to register the position of the robot. Planning software is used for organ segmentation and defining the needle path. Dose constraints and organ contours are used by the planning software to determine the optimal location for the seeds. Needle penetration and source delivery are automated and controlled remotely by the surgeon [139]. This system was experimentally tested in 4 male dogs for prostate brachytherapy [140]. Results showed a mean placement error of the seeds of 3.32±2.77 mm.

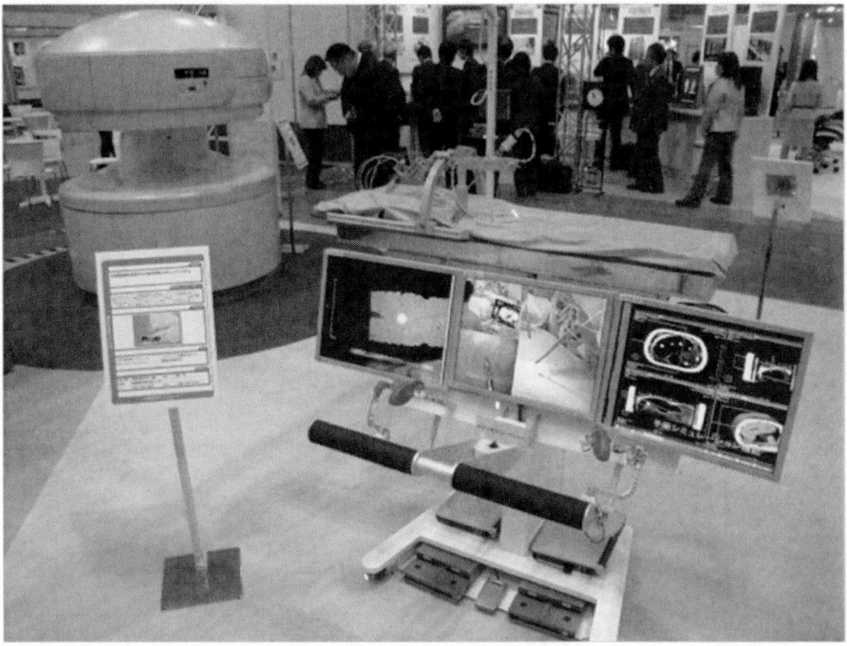

Figure 7. MRI-guided surgical robotic system. The photograph shows an open-bone MR scanner in the top left, the MRI-compatible operating table with the compact MRI-compatible surgical manipulator (slave) in the upper right, and the surgical console with the manipulator (master) at the bottom (Courtesy of Prof. M. Hashizume, Department of Advanced Medical Initiatives, Kyushu University, Fukuoka, Japan).

Conclusion

The introduction of computer-assisted surgery, including image-guided surgery and robot-assisted surgery, to support surgical interventions has provided surgeons with new assistance tools to address some limitations of MIS as well as improve the clinical outcomes. In general terms, the magnified operative field and the increased surgical dexterity result in a low conversion rate and reduced tissue trauma. With improved computer and imaging technologies, navigation systems are quickly becoming an integral part in the surgical routine in hospitals. These systems improve the surgeon perception of the patient anatomy and provide tools to analyze in advance the most suited approach to carry out a surgical intervention. In this sense, AR offers a suitable way to enhance the common view of the surgical field with useful information as preoperative images and virtual models. Although this technology is well established for rigid anatomy, further work has to be done for a full integration with deformable anatomical models. Continuous technological advances in robotic-assisted surgery have led to potential improvements in the development of MIS procedures such as 3D vision, increased precision and dexterity, and ergonomic conditions for the surgeon. Besides, novel robotic prototypes are being developed for recent MIS approaches such as LESS and NOTES. New dexterous and micro-robotic systems are able to enter the body via a LESS or NOTES approach, providing assistance during the surgical intervention. However, there is currently no ideal platform for these surgeries. Each kind of procedure may require a customized solution to provide a feasible surgical robotic system.

References

[1] Galloway R, Peters T. *Overview and History of Image-Guided Interventions.* In: Image-guided interventions: technology and applications. 2008. Springer New York.

[2] Jolesz FA. Introduction. In: Intraoperative Imaging and Image- Guided Therapy. Jolesz FA, editor. 2014. Springer New York.

[3] Kapur T, Egger J, Jayender J, Toews M, Wells WM. Registration and Segmentation for Image-Guided Therapy. In: *Intraoperative Imaging and Image- Guided Therapy.* Jolesz FA, editor. 2014. Springer New York.

[4] Cleary K, Wilson E, Ordas S, Banovac F. Navigation. In: *Intraoperative Imaging and Image- Guided Therapy.* Jolesz FA, editor. 2014. Springer New York.

[5] Sánchez-Margallo JA, Sánchez-Margallo FM, Oropesa I, Gómez EJ. Systems and technologies for objective evaluation of technical skills in laparoscopic surgery. *Minim Invasive Ther Allied Technol* 2014;23(1):40–51.

[6] Sugimoto M, Yasuda H, Koda K, Suzuki M, Yamazaki M, Tezuka T, et al. Image overlay navigation by markerless surface registration in gastrointestinal, hepatobiliary and pancreatic surgery. *J Hepatobiliary Pancreat Sci.* 2010;17:629–36.

[7] Oguro S, Tokuda J, Elhawary H, Haker S, Kikinis R, Tempany CM, Hata N. MRI signal intensity based B-spline nonrigid registration for pre- and intraoperative imaging during prostate brachytherapy. *J Magn Reson Imaging* 2009;30(5):1052–8.

[8] Archip N, Tatli S, Morrison P, Jolesz F, Warfi eld SK, Silverman S. Non-rigid registration of pre-procedural MR images with intra-procedural unenhanced CT images for improved targeting of tumors during liver radiofrequency ablations. *Med Image Comput Comput Assist Interv* 2007;10(Pt 2):969–77.

[9] Teber D, Guven S, Simpfendörfer T, Baumhauer M, Güven EO, Yencilek F, Gözen AS, Rassweiler J. Augmented reality: a new tool to improve surgical accuracy during laparoscopic partial nephrectomy? Preliminary in vitro and in vivo results. *Eur Urol* 2009;56(2):332-8.

[10] Shekhar R, Dandekar O, Bhat V, Philip M, Lei P, Godinez C, et al. Live augmented reality: a new visualization method for laparoscopic surgery using continuous volumetric computed tomography. *Surg Endosc* 2010;24(8):1976–85.

[11] Okamoto T, Onda S, Yanaga K, Suzuki N, Hattori A. Clinical application of navigation surgery using augmented reality in the abdominal field. Surg Today 2014. [Epub ahead of print].

[12] Pieper SD. Visualization and Display for Image-Guided Therapy. In: *Intraoperative Imaging and Image- Guided Therapy.* Jolesz FA, editor. 2014. Springer New York.

[13] Liao H, Inomata T, Sakuma I, Dohi T. 3-D augmented reality for MRI-guided surgery using integral videography autostereoscopic image overlay. *IEEE Trans Biomed Eng* 2010;57(6):1476–86.

[14] Soler L, Nicolau S, Pessaux P, Mutter D, Marescaux J. Real-time 3D image reconstruction guidance in liver resection surgery. *Hepatobiliary Surg Nutr* 2014;3(2):73–81.

[15] Soler L, Forest C, Nicolau S, Vayssiere C, Wattiez A, Marescaux J. Computer-assisted operative procedure: from preoperative planning to simulation. *Eur Clin Obstet Gynaecol* 2006;2(4):201–8.

[16] Gering DT, Nabavi a, Kikinis R, Hata N, O'Donnell LJ, Grimson WE, et al. An integrated visualization system for surgical planning and guidance using image fusion and an open MR. *J Magn Reson Imaging* 2001;13(6):967–75.

[17] Ferroli P, Tringali G, Acerbi F, Schiariti M, Broggi M, Aquino D, Broggi G (2013) Advanced 3-dimensional planning in neurosurgery. *Neurosurg Suppl* 1:A54–A62.

[18] Stelter K, Ertl-Wagner B, Luz M, Muller S, Ledderose G, Siedek V, Berghaus A, Arpe S, Leunig A. Evaluation of an image-guided navigation system in the training of functional endoscopic sinus surgeons. A prospective, randomised clinical study. *Rhinology* 2011;49(4):429-37.

[19] Wilson DA, Astephen Wilson JL, Richardson G, Dunbar MJ. Changes in the functional flexion axis of the knee before and after total knee arthroplasty using a navigation system. *J Arthroplasty* 2014;29(7):1388-93

[20] Hong J, Matsumoto N, Ouchida R, Komune S, Hashizume M. Medical navigation system for otologic surgery based on hybrid registration and virtual intraoperative computed tomography. *IEEE Trans Biomed Eng* 2009;56(2):426–432.

[21] Mezger U, Jendrewski C, Bartels M. Navigation in surgery. *Langenbecks Arch Surg.* 2013;398:501–14.

[22] Wood BJ, Kruecker J, Abi-Jaoudeh N, Locklin JK, Levy E, Xu S et al. Navigation systems for ablation. *J Vasc Interv Radiol.* 2010;21(8):S257–63.

[23] Beyar R. Navigation within the heart and vessels in clinical prac-tice. *Ann N Y Acad Sci.* 2010;1188(1):207–13.

[24] Baumhauer M, Feuerstein M, Meinzer HP et al. Navigation in endoscopic soft tissue surgery: perspectives and limitations. *J Endourol* 2008;22:751–766.

[25] Ukimura O, Gill IS (2008) Imaging-assisted endoscopic surgery: cleveland clinic experience. *J Endourol* 22:803–810.

[26] Birkfellner W, Hummel J, Wilson E, Cleary K. Tracking Devices. In: Peters T, Cleary K, editors. *Image-guided interventions: technology and applications.* Springer New York; 2008.

[27] Micali S, Pini G, Teber D. New trends in minimally invasive urological surgery. What is beyond the robot?. *World J Urol* 2013;31(3):505–13.

[28] Marescaux J, Rubino F, Arenas M, Mutter D, Soler L. Augmented-reality-assisted laparoscopic adrenalectomy. *JAMA* 2004;292:2214–5.

[29] Tsutsumi N, Tomikawa M, Uemura M, Akahoshi T, Nagao Y, Konishi K, et al. Image-guided laparoscopic surgery in an open MRI operating theater. *Surg Endosc* 2013;27(6):2178–84.

[30] Simpfendörfer T, Baumhauer M, Müller M, Gutt CN, Meinzer HP, Rassweiler JJ, et al. Augmented reality visualization during laparoscopic radical prostatectomy. *J Endourol.* 2011;25:1841–5.

[31] Ieiri S, Uemura M, Konishi K, Souzaki R, Nagao Y, Tsutsumi N, et al. Augmented reality navigation system for laparoscopic splenectomy in children based on preoperative CT image using optical tracking device. *Pediatr Surg Int* 2012;28(4):341–6.

[32] Vahrmeijer AL, Hutteman M, van der Vorst JR, van de Velde CJ, Frangioni JV. Image-guided cancer surgery using near-infrared fluorescence. *Nat Rev Clin Oncol* 2013;10(9):507-18.

[33] Nguyen QT, Tsien RY. Fluorescence-guided surgery with live molecular navigation--a new cutting edge. *Nat Rev Cancer* 2013;13(9):653–62.

[34] Kudo H, Ishizawa T, Tani K, Harada N, Ichida A, Shimizu A, et al. Visualization of subcapsular hepatic malignancy by indocyanine-green fluorescence imaging during laparoscopic hepatectomy. *Surg Endosc* 2014;28(8):2504–8.

[35] Diana M, Noll E, Diemunsch P, Dallemagne B, Benahmed M a, Agnus V, et al. Enhanced-reality video fluorescence: a real-time assessment of intestinal viability. *Ann Surg* 2014;259(4):700–7.

[36] Mohsen A, Elbasiouny MS, Fawzy YS. Fluorescence-guided laparoscopic cholecystectomy: a new technique for visualization of biliary system by using fluorescein. *Surg Innov* 2013;20(2):105–8.

[37] Schols RM, Lodewick TM, Bouvy ND, van Dam DA, Meijerink WJ, van Dam GM, Dejong CH, Stassen LP. Near-infrared fluorescence laparoscopy of the cystic duct and artery in pigs: performance of a preclinical dye. *J Laparoendosc Adv Surg Tech A* 2014;24(5):318-22.

[38] Kondo Y, Murayama Y, Konishi H, Morimura R, Komatsu S, Shiozaki A, et al. Fluorescent detection of peritoneal metastasis in human

colorectal cancer using 5-aminolevulinic acid. *Int J Oncol* 2014;45(1):41–6.

[39] Jichlinski P, Forrer M, Mizeret J, Glanzmann T, Braichotte D, Wagnieres G, Zimmer G, Guillou L, Schmidlin F, Graber P, van den Bergh H and Leisinger HJ: Clinical evaluation of a method for detecting superficial surgical transitional cell carcinoma of the bladder by light induced fluorescence of protoporphyrin IX following the topical application of 5-aminolevulinic acid: preliminary results. *Lasers Surg Med* 1997;20: 402-408.

[40] Friesen SA, Hjortland GO, Madsen SJ, Hirschberg H, Engebraten O, Nesland JM and Peng Q: 5-Aminolevulinic acid-based photo-dynamic detection and therapy of brain tumors (review). *Int J Oncol* 2002;21: 577-582.

[41] Hoda MR, Popken G. Surgical outcomes of fluorescence-guided laparoscopic partial nephrectomy using 5-aminolevulinic acid-induced protoporphyrin IX. *J Surg Res* 2009;154(2):220–5.

[42] Tobis S, Knopf JK, Silvers C, Messing E, Yao J, Rashid H, et al. Robot-assisted and laparoscopic partial nephrectomy with near infrared fluorescence imaging. *J Endourol* 2012;26(7):797–802.

[43] Hockenberry MS, Smith ZL, Mucksavage P. A novel use of near-infrared fluorescence imaging during robotic surgery without contrast agents. *J Endourol* 2014;28(5):509-12.

[44] Ohuchida K, Hashizume M. Overview of Robotic Surgery. In: Watanabe G, editor. Robotic Surgery. Tokyo: Springer Japan; 2014.

[45] Benabid AL, Cinquin P, Lavalle S, Le Bas JF, Demongeot J, de Rougemont J. Computer-driven robot for stereotactic surgery connected to CT scan and magnetic resonance imaging. Technological design and preliminary results. *Appl Neurophysiol* 1987; 50:153–154.

[46] Kwoh YS, Hou J, Jonckheere EA, Hayati S. A robot with improved absolute positioning accuracy for CT guided stereotactic brain surgery. *IEEE Trans Biomed Eng* 1988; 35:153–160.

[47] Wedmid A, Llukani E, Lee DI. Future perspectives in robotic surgery. *BJU Int* 2011;108(6 Pt 2):1028–36.

[48] Mettler L, Ibrahim M, Jonat W. One year of experience working with the aid of a robotic assistant (the voice-controlled optic holder AESOP) in gynaecological endoscopic surgery. *Hum Reprod* 1998;13(1O):2748-50.

[49] Wagner AA, Varkarakis IM, Link RE, Sullivan W, Su LM. Comparison of surgical performance during laparoscopic radical prostatectomy of

two robotic camera holders, EndoAssist and AESOP: a pilot study. *Urology* 2006;68(1):70-4.

[50] Ewing DR, Pigazzi a., Wang Y, Ballantyne GH. Robots in the Operating Room The History. *Surg Innov* 2004;11(2):63–71.

[51] Satava RM. Robotic surgery: from past to future: a personal journey. *Surg Clin North Am* 2003; 83:1491–1500.

[52] Kiaii B, Boyd WD, Rayman R, et al. Robot-assisted computer enhanced closed-chest coronary surgery: preliminary experience using a harmonic scalpel and Zeus. *Heart Surg Forum* 2000;3:194-197.

[53] Boehm DH, Reichenspurner H, Detter C, et al. Clinical use of a computer-enhanced surgical robotic system for endoscopic coronary artery bypass grafting on the beating heart. *J Thorac Cardiovasc Surg* 2000;48:198-202.

[54] Marescaux J, Leroy J, Gagner M, Rubino F, Mutter D, Vix M et al. Transatlantic robot- assisted telesurgery. *Nature* 2001; 413(6854):379–380.

[55] Satava RM. Surgical robotics: the early chronicles: a personal historical perspective. *Surg Laparosc Endosc Percutan Tech* 2002; 12:6–16.

[56] Hagen ME, Curet MJ. The da Vinci Surgical® Systems. In: Watanabe G, editor. Robotic Surgery. Tokyo: Springer Japan; 2014.

[57] Hagen ME, Pugin F, Chassot G, Huber O, Buchs N, Iranmanesh P, Morel P. Reducing cost of surgery by avoiding complications: the model of robotic Roux-en-Y gastric bypass. *Obes Surg* 2012; 22(1):52–61.

[58] Augustin F, Bodner J, Wykypiel H, Schwinghammer C, Schmid T. Perioperative results of robotic lung lobectomy: summary of literature. *Surg Endosc* 2012; 26:1190–1191.

[59] Morel P, Buchs NC, Iranmanesh P, Pugin F, Buehler L, Azagury DE, Jung M, Volonte F, Hagen ME. Robotic single-site cholecystectomy. *J Hepatobiliary Pancreat Sci* 2014;21(1):18-25.

[60] Tobis S, Houman J, Thomer M, Rashid H, Wu G. Robot-assisted transumbilical laparoendoscopic single-site pyeloplasty: technique and perioperative outcomes from a single institution. *J Laparoendosc Adv Surg Tech A* 2013;23(8):702-6.

[61] Laydner H, Autorino R, Isac W, Khalifeh A, Panumatrassamee K, Kassab A, et al. Robotic retroperitoneal transvaginal natural orifice translumenal endoscopic surgery (NOTES) nephrectomy: feasibility study in a cadaver model. *Urology* 2013;81(6):1232–7.

[62] Eyraud R, Laydner H, Autorino R, Hillyer S, Long J-A, Panumatrassamee K, et al. Robot-assisted transrectal hybrid natural

orifice translumenal endoscopic surgery nephrectomy and adrenalectomy: initial investigation in a cadaver model. *Urology* 2013;81(5):1090–4.

[63] Olanrewaju OA, Faieza AA, Syakirah K. Current trend of robotics application in medical. In: *IOP Conference Series: Materials Science and Engineering. Vol.* 46. IOP Publishing. 2013.

[64] Connor S, Garden OJ. Bile duct injury in the era of laparoscopic cholecystectomy. *Br J Surg* 2006; 93:158–168.

[65] Bann S, Khan M, Hernandez J, Munz Y, Moorthy K, Datta V, et al. Robotics in surgery. *J Am Coll Surg* 2003;196(5):784–95.

[66] Autorino R, Zargar H, Kaouk JH. *Robotic-assisted laparoscopic surgery: recent advances in urology.* Fertil Steril 2014 [Epub ahead of print].

[67] Tachibana M, Yoshioka K. Robotic Surgery in Urology. In: Watanabe G, editor. *Robotic Surgery.* Tokyo: Springer Japan; 2014.

[68] Schuessler WW, Schulam PG, Clayman RV, Kavoussi LR. Laparoscopic radical prostatectomy: initial short-term experience. *Urology* 1997; 50(6):854–857.

[69] Krambeck AE, DiMarco DS, Rangel LJ, Bergstralh EJ, Blute ML, Gettman MT. Radical prostatectomy for prostatic adenocarcinoma: a matched comparison of open retropubic and robot-assisted techniques. *BJU Int* 2009; 103(4):448–453.

[70] Richards KA, Hemal AK, Kader AK, Pettus JA. Robot assisted laparoscopic pelvic lymphadenectomy at the time of radical cystectomy rivals that of open surgery: single institution report. *Urology* 2010; 76:1400–1404.

[71] Coelho RF, Rocco B, Patel MB, Orvieto MA, Chauhan S, Ficarra V et al. Retropubic, laparoscopic, and robot-assisted radical prostatectomy: a critical review of outcomes reported by high-volume centers. *J Endourol* 2010; 24:2003–2015

[72] Orvieto MA, Patel VR. Evolution of robot-assisted radical prostatectomy. *Scand J Surg* 2009; 98(2):76–88.

[73] Hanzly M, Fredrick A, Creighton T, Attwood K, Mehedint D, Kauffman E, Kim HL, Schwaab T. Learning Curves for Robotic-Assisted and Laparoscopic Partial Nephrectomy. *J Endourol* 2014;11 [Epub ahead of print].

[74] Gettman MT, Blute ML, Chow GK, Neururer R, Bartsch G, Peschel R. Robotic-assisted laparoscopic partial nephrectomy: technique and initial

clinical experience with daVinci robotic system. *Urology* 2004; 64:914–918.

[75] Brandina R, Aron M. Laparoscopic partial nephrectomy: advances since 2005. *Curr Opin Urol* 2010; 20:111–118.

[76] Haseebuddin M, Benway BM, Cabello JM, Bhayani SB. Robot-assisted partial nephrec- tomy: evaluation of learning curve for an experienced renal surgeon. *J Endourol* 2010; 24:57–61.

[77] Stephenson ER, Sankholkar S, Ducko CT, Damiano RJ. Robotically assisted microsurgery for endoscopic coronary artery bypass grafting. *Ann Thorac Surg* 1998; 66:1064–1067.

[78] Loulmet D, Carpentier A, d' Attelis N et al. Endoscopic coronary artery bypass grafting with the aid of computer-assisted instruments. *J Thorac Cardiovasc Surg* 1999;48:4–10.

[79] Carpentier A, Loulmet D, Aupècle B, et al. Computer assisted open heart surgery. First case operated on with success. *C R Acad Sci III* 1998;321:437-42

[80] Chi NH, Huang CH, Huang SC, Yu HY, Chen YS, Wang SS, Wu IH. Robotic mitral valve repair in infective endocarditis. *J Thorac Dis* 2014;6(1):56-60.

[81] Srivastava S, Gadasalli S, Agusala M, Kolluru R, Naidu J, Shroff M, Barrera R, Quismundo S, Srivastava V. Use of bilateral internal thoracic arteries in CABG through lateral thoracotomy with robotic assistance in 150 patients. *Ann Thorac Surg* 2006; 81:800–806.

[82] Watanabe G. Cardiac Surgery: Overview. In: Watanabe G, editor. Robotic Surgery. Tokyo: Springer Japan; 2014.

[83] Robicsek F. Robotic cardiac surgery: time told! *J Thorac Cardiovasc Surg* 2008;135:243–246.

[84] Ota T, Degani A, Schwartzman D, Zubiate B, McGarvey J, Choset H, Zenati MA. A highly articulated robotic surgical system for minimally invasive surgery. *Ann Thorac Surg* 2009; 87:1253–1256.

[85] Lee HS, Jang HJ. Robotic Surgery in General Thoracic Surgery. In: Watanabe G, editor. Robotic Surgery. Tokyo: Springer Japan; 2014.

[86] Nasir BS, Bryant AS, Minnich DJ, Wei B, Cerfolio RJ. Performing robotic lobectomy and segmentectomy: cost, profitability, and outcomes. *Ann Thorac Surg* 2014;98(1):203-8; discussion 208-9.

[87] Melfi FM, Fanucchi O, Davini F, Romano G, Lucchi M, Dini P, Ambrogi MC, Mussi A. Robotic lobectomy for lung cancer: evolution in technique and technology. *Eur J Cardiothorac Surg* 2014;9 [Epub ahead of print].

[88] Jang HJ, Lee HS, Park SY, Zo JI. Comparison of the early robot-assisted lobectomy experience to video-assisted thoracic surgery lobectomy for lung cancer: a single-institution case series matching study. *Innovations* 2011; 6(5):305–310.

[89] Park BJ, Flores RM. Cost comparison of robotic, video-assisted thoracic surgery and thoracotomy approaches to pulmonary lobectomy. *Thorac Surg Clin* 2008;18(3):297–300.

[90] Toker A, Erus S, Ozkan B, Ziyade S, Tanju S. Does a relationship exist between the number of thoracoscopic thymectomies performed and the learning curve for thoracoscopic resection of thymoma in patients with myasthenia gravis? *Interact Cardiovasc Thorac Surg* 2011; 12 (2):152–155.

[91] Díaz-Montes TP, Tanner EJ, Fader AN. Instrumentation, Platforms, and Basic Principles of Robotics. In: Escobar P, Falcone T, editors. *Atlas of Single-Port, Laparoscopic, and Robotic Surgery.* Springer New York; 2014.

[92] Magrina JF, Zanagnolo V, Giles D, Noble BN, Kho RM, Magtibay PM. Robotic surgery for endometrial cancer: comparison of perioperative outcomes and recurrence with laparoscopy, vaginal/laparoscopy and laparotomy. *Eur J Gynaecol Oncol* 2011;32:476–80.

[93] Orady M. Robotic-Assisted Total Laparoscopic Hysterectomy. In: Escobar P, Falcone T, editors. *Atlas of Single-Port, Laparoscopic, and Robotic Surgery.* Springer New York; 2014.

[94] Magrina JF, Kho R, Magtibay PM. Robotic radi- cal hysterectomy: technical aspects. *Gynecol Oncol* 2009;113:28–31.

[95] Hsiao SM, Lin HH, Peng FS, Jen PJ, Hsiao CF, Tu FC. Comparison of robot-assisted laparoscopic myomectomy and traditional laparoscopic myomectomy. *J Obstet Gynaecol Res* 2013;39(5):1024-9.

[96] Holloway RW, Bravo RA, Rakowski JA, James JA, Jeppson CN, Ingersoll SB, Ahmad S. Detection of sentinel lymph nodes in patients with endometrial cancer undergoing robotic-assisted staging: a comparison of colorimetric and fluorescence imaging. *Gynecol Oncol.* 2012;126(1):25-9.

[97] Emami CN, Garrett D, Anselmo D, Nguyen NX. Pediatric single incision laparoscopic cholecystectomy: lessons learned in the first 25 cases. *Pediatr Surg Int* 2011; 27:743–746.

[98] Park HS, Kim TJ, Song T, Kim MK, Lee YY, Choi CH, Lee JW, Kim BG, Bae DS. Single-port access (SPA) laparoscopic surgery in

gynecology: a surgeon's experience with an initial 200 cases. *Eur J Obstet Gynecol Reprod Biol* 2011; 154:81–84

[99] Gaujoux S, Kingham TP, Jarnagin WR, D'Angelica MI, Allen PJ, Fong Y. Single-incision laparoscopic liver resection. *Surg Endosc* 2011; 25:1489–1494.

[100] White MA, Haber G-P, Kaouk JH. Robotic single-site surgery. *Curr Opin Urol* 2010; 20(1): 86-91.

[101] Islam A, Castellvi AO, Tesfay ST, Castellvi AD, Wright AS, Scott DJ. Early surgeon impressions and technical diffi- culty associated with laparoendoscopic single-site surgery: a Society of American Gastrointestinal and Endoscopic Surgeons learning center study. *Surg Endosc* 2011; 25:2597–2603.

[102] Pérez-Duarte FJ, Lucas-Hernández M, Matos-Azevedo A, Sánchez-Margallo JA, Díaz-Güemes I, Sánchez-Margallo FM. Objective analysis of surgeons' ergonomy during laparoendoscopic single-site surgery through the use of surface electromyography and a motion capture data glove. *Surg Endosc* 2014;28(4):1314–20.

[103] Escobar PF, Fader AN, Paraiso MF, Kaouk JH, Falcone T. Robotic-assisted laparoendoscopic single- site sur- gery in gynecology: initial report and technique. *J Minim Invasive Gynecol* 2009;16:589–91.

[104] Kaouk JH, Goel RK, Haber GP, Crouzet S, Stein RJ. Robotic single-port transumbilical surgery in humans: initial report. *BJU Int* 2009; 103(3):366–369.

[105] White WM, Haber G-P, Goel RK, et al. Single-port urological surgery: single-center experience with the first 100 cases. *Urology* 2009 Oct; 74(4): 801–804.

[106] Ostrowitz MB, Eschete D, Zemon H, DeNoto G. Robotic-assisted single-incision right colectomy: early experience. *Int J Med Robot* 2009 Dec; 5(4): 465–470.

[107] Romanelli JR, Roshek TB 3rd, Lynn DC, Earle DB. Single-port laparoscopic cholecystectomy: initial experience. *Surg Endosc* 2010 Jun; 24(6): 1374–1379.

[108] Allemann P, Leroy J, Asakuma M, et al. Robotics may overcome technical limitations of single-trocar surgery. *Arch Surg* 2010 Mar; 145(3): 267–271.

[109] Haber G-P, White MA, Autorino R, et al. Novel robotic da Vinci instruments for laparoendoscopic single-site surgery. *Urology* 2010 Dec; 76(6): 1279–1282.

[110] Petroni G, Niccolini M, Menciassi A, Dario P, Cuschieri A. A novel intracorporeal assembling robotic system for single-port laparoscopic surgery. *Surg Endosc* 2013;27(2):665–70.

[111] Petroni G, Niccolini M, Caccavaro S, Quaglia C, Menciassi A, Schostek S, et al. A novel robotic system for single-port laparoscopic surgery: preliminary experience. *Surg Endosc* 2013;27(6):1932–7.

[112] Cheon B, Gezgin E, Ji DK, Tomikawa M, Hashizume M, Kim H-J, et al. A single port laparoscopic surgery robot with high force transmission and a large workspace. *Surg Endosc* 2014;28(9):2719–29.

[113] Sanchez-Margallo FM, Perez FJ, Sanchez MA, Asencio JM, del Carmen Tejonero M, Moreno C, Noguera J. Hybrid notes cholecystectomy in an experimental model of laparoscopic acute cholecystitis. *Surg Laparosc Endosc Percutan Tech* 2011;21(2):e65-9.

[114] Noguera JF, Cuadrado A, Sánchez-Margallo FM, Dolz C, Asencio JM, Olea JM, Morales R, Lozano L, Vicens JC. Emergency transvaginal hybrid natural orifice transluminal endoscopic surgery. *Endoscopy* 2011;43(5):442-4.

[115] Bulian DR, Runkel N, Burghardt J, Lamade W, Butters M, Utech M, Thon KP, Lefering R, Heiss MM, Buhr HJ, Lehmann KS. Natural Orifice Transluminal Endoscopic Surgery (NOTES) for colon resections--analysis of the first 139 patients of the German NOTES Registry (GNR). *Int J Colorectal Dis* 2014;29(7):853-61.

[116] Haber GP, Crouzet S, Kamoi K, Berger A, Aron M, Goel R et al. Robotic NOTES (natural orifice translumenal endoscopic surgery) in reconstructive urology: initial laboratory experience. *Urology* 2008; 71:996–1000.

[117] Demura Y, Ishikawa N, Hirano Y, Inaki N, Matsunoki A, Watanabe G. Transrectal robotic natural orifice translumenal endoscopic surgery (NOTES) applied to intestinal anastomosis in a porcine intestine model. *Surg Endosc* 2013;27(12):4693–701.

[118] Suzuki N, Hattori A, Ieiri S, Konishi K, Maeda T, Fujino Y, et al. Telecontrol of an endoscopic surgical robot system between Japan and Thailand for tele-NOTES. *Stud Health Technol Inform* 2009;142:374–9.

[119] Spaun GO, Zheng B, Swanström LL. A multitasking platform for natural orifice translumenal endoscopic surgery (NOTES): a benchtop comparison of a new device for flexible endoscopic surgery and a standard dual-channel endoscope. *Surg Endosc* 2009;2720–7.

[120] Fuchs K-H, Breithaupt W. Transgastric small bowel resection with the new multitasking platform EndoSAMURAI™ for natural orifice transluminal endoscopic surgery. *Surg Endosc* 2012;26(8):2281–7.

[121] Phee SJ, Low SC, Huynh V a, Kencana a P, Sun ZL, Yang K. Master and slave transluminal endoscopic robot (MASTER) for natural orifice transluminal endoscopic surgery (NOTES). Conf. Proc. *IEEE Eng Med Biol Soc* 2009;1192–5.

[122] Phee SJ, Reddy N, Chiu PWY, Rebala P, Rao G V, Wang Z, et al. Robot-assisted endoscopic submucosal dissection is effective in treating patients with early-stage gastric neoplasia. *Clin Gastroenterol Hepatol* 2012;10(10):1117–21.

[123] Phee SJ, Ho KY, Lomanto D, Low SC, Huynh V a, Kencana a P, et al. Natural orifice transgastric endoscopic wedge hepatic resection in an experimental model using an intuitively controlled master and slave transluminal endoscopic robot (MASTER). *Surg Endosc* 2010;24(9):2293–8.

[124] Yeung BPM, Gourlay T. A technical review of flexible endoscopic multitasking platforms. *Int J Surg* 2012;10(7):345–54.

[125] Lehman AC, Dumpert J, Wood N a, Redden L, Visty AQ, Farritor S, et al. Natural orifice cholecystectomy using a miniature robot. *Surg Endosc* 2009;23(2):260–6.

[126] Dieterich S, Gibbs IC. The CyberKnife in clinical use: current roles, future expectations. *Front Radiat Ther Oncol* 2011;43:181–94.

[127] Adler JR Jr, Chang SD, Murphy MJ, Doty J, Geis P, Hancock SL. The Cyberknife: a frameless robotic system for radiosurgery. *Stereotact Funct Neurosurg* 1997; 69:124–128.

[128] Adler JR Jr, Murphy MJ, Chang SD, Hancock SL. Image-guided robotic radiosurgery. *Neurosurgery* 1999; 44:1299–1306, Discussion 1306-7.

[129] Koethe Y, Xu S, Velusamy G, Wood BJ, Venkatesan AM. Accuracy and efficacy of percutaneous biopsy and ablation using robotic assistance under computed tomography guidance: a phantom study. *Eur Radiol* 2014;24(3):723–30.

[130] Abdullah BJ, Yeong CH, Goh K, Yoong B, Ho G, Kulkarni A. Early experience of a commercial available robot (Maxio) for CT-guided radiofrequency ablation of liver tumours. *Insights Imaging* (2014) 5 (Suppl 1):S162.

[131] Di Biase L, Natale A, Barrett C, Tan C, Elayi CS, Ching CK, et al. Relationship between catheter forces, lesion characteristics, "popping,"

and char formation: experience with robotic navigation system. *J Cardiovasc Electrophysiol* 2009;20(4):436-40.

[132] Hlivák P, Mlčochová H, Peichl P, Cihák R, Wichterle D, Kautzner J. Robotic navigation in catheter ablation for paroxysmal atrial fibrillation: midterm efficacy and predictors of postablation arrhythmia recurrences. *J Cardiovasc Electrophysiol* 2011;22(5):534-40.

[133] Thomas D, Scholz EP, Schweizer PA, Katus HA, Becker R. Initial experience with robotic navigation for catheter ablation of paroxysmal and persistent atrial fibrillation. *J Electrocardiol* 2012;45(2):95-101.

[134] Steven D, Servatius H, Rostock T, Hoffmann B, Drewitz I, Müllerleile K, Sultan A, Aydin MA, Meinertz T, Willems S. Reduced fluoroscopy during atrial fibrillation ablation: benefits of robotic guided navigation. *J Cardiovasc Electrophysiol* 2010;21(1):6-12.

[135] Schmidt B, Chun KRJ, Tilz RR, Koektuerk B, Ouyang F, Kuck K-H. Remote navigation systems in electrophysiology. *Europace* 2008;10(Suppl 3):iii57–61.

[136] Arya A, Zaker-Shahrak R, Sommer P, Bollmann A, Wetzel U, Gaspar T, et al. Catheter ablation of atrial fibrillation using remote magnetic catheter navigation: a case–control study. *Europace* 2011;13:45–50.

[137] Lüthje L, Vollmann D, Seegers J, Dorenkamp M, Sohns C. Hasenfuss Get al. Remote magnetic versus manual catheter navigation for circumferential pulmonary vein ablation in patients with atrial fibrillation. *Clinical Research in Cardiology* 2011;100:1003–1011.

[138] Hashizume M, Yasunaga T, Tanoue K, Ieiri S, Konishi K, Kishi K, et al. New real-time MR image-guided surgical robotic system for minimally invasive precision surgery. *Int J Comput Assist Radiol Surg* 2008;2(6):317–25.

[139] Cunha JA, Hsu I-C, Pouliot J, Roach Iii M, Shinohara K, Kurhanewicz J, et al. Toward adaptive stereotactic robotic brachytherapy for prostate cancer: demonstration of an adaptive workflow incorporating inverse planning and an MR stealth robot. *Minim Invasive Ther Allied Technol* 2010;19(4):189–202.

[140] Stoianovici D, Song DY, Petrisor D, Mozer P, Armour E, Vigaru B, Muntener M, Patriciu A, Schar M. MRI-compatible pneumatic robot (MRBot) for prostate brachytherapy: Preclinical assessment of accuracy and execution of dosimetric plans. *International Journal of Radiation Oncology* Biology* Physics* 2008;72(1):S306-S307.

In: Computer-Assisted Surgery
Editor: Xiaojun Chen

ISBN: 978-1-63463-811-1

Chapter 4

MODIFIED METHODS OF SETTING UP THE SPINAL NAVIGATION SYSTEM

Sang Hoon Jang* and Ho-Yeon Lee
Department of Neurosurgery,
Gang-buk Wooridul Spine Hospital, Seoul, Korea

ABSTRACT

There are many reports about accuracy and efficacy of the spinal navigation system but most of their topics are limited to spinal instrumentation. For minimally invasive surgery, important things are how to set up navigation system fast and efficiently without interference of surgical flow, and how to use the navigation system within a small working field. Our team has already introduced a skin fixed dynamic reference frame (DRF) into mini open transforaminal lumbar interbody fusion (TLIF) and recently examined the accuracy of skin-fixed DRF in the anterior cervical foraminotomy. Both methods require only few minutes to set up and do not prohibit the natural movement of the surgeon during the operation. We want to share detailed methods about setting up the navigation system and the knowhow of using navigation systems, especially in minimally invasive spinal surgeries.

Keywords: Spinal navigation system, skin fixed dynamic reference frame

---

* Correspondence to: Email: iamleesol@gmail.com.

1. Introduction

Recently a number of different manufacturers offer spinal navigation systems, which utilize preoperative CT scans to intraoperative 3D images, which are widely used in spinal surgeries [1-5]. Although there are some differences in hardware and software functions, these systems basically enable surgical instruments to be shown in reference to the displayed imaging anatomy in real time. Therefore, a more precise and delicate operation, after minimal exposure of the spinal structures could even be possible in deformed or severely degenerated spines [6]. There is a steep learning curve in using the navigation system, which is difficult and requires a significant amount of time, especially in the case of early experience of image guided surgery, even in a simple procedure [3-5]. Among every step of introducing the navigation system, the most important thing is the registration process for matching the image anatomy to the surgical anatomy. Setting reliable reference frames have an important role in reducing registration inaccuracy. Usually, setting up the navigation system is done with the fixed reference frame (FRF), which is attached to a head rest or operation table. But in this circumstance, the positioning change of the patient, on the operation table, can cause significant errors in the navigation system.

A dynamic reference frame (DRF) is firmly attached to the patient's body, which helps to overcome these weak-points. Bone fixed DRF usually requires another separate skin incision, or a longer incision, and occasionally interferes surgeon's movement. Skin fixed DRF can be a solution to these problems, and are designed as a fast and efficient method for minimal invasive surgery without interference of surgical flow and within a small working field.

2. Materials and Methods

2.1. Indication

- Minimal invasive anterior foraminotomy in cervical spine
- Multilevel oblique corpectomy of cervical spine in case of ossified posterior longitudinal ligament (OPLL) or cervical spondylotic myelopathy (CSM)
- Minimal invasive posterior cervical foraminotomy
- Posterior cervical instrumentation

- Thoracic posterior decompression surgery using a tubular retractor
- Pedicle screw insertion in thoracic spine
- Paraspinal decompression for extraforaminal lumbar disc herniation,
- Mini open transforaminal lumbar interbody fusion (TLIF).

2.2. Instrumentations

– Cone beam CT (O arm® Medtronic Sofamor Danek, Memphis, TN) (Figure 1).

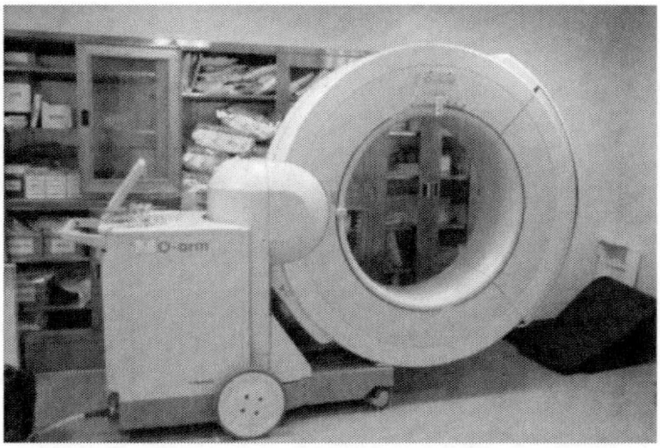

Figure 1. Cone beam CT(O arm® Medtronic Sofamor Danek, Memphis, TN).

– Navigation system (Stealthstation® Medtronic Sofamor Danek, Memphis, TN) (Figure 2).

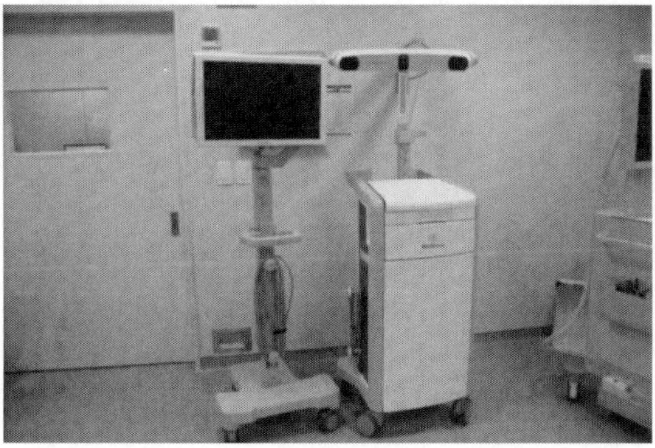

Figure 2. Navigation system (Stealthstation® Medtronic Sofamor Danek, Memphis, TN).

– Incised surgical film (OPSITE® Smith & Nephew, Hull, UK) (Figure 3).

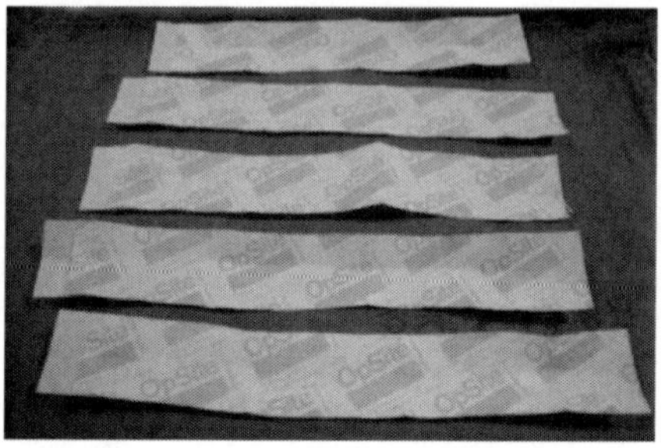

Figure 3. Incised surgical film (OPSITE® Smith & Nephew, Hull, UK).

– Dynamic reference frame (DRF) (Figure 4).

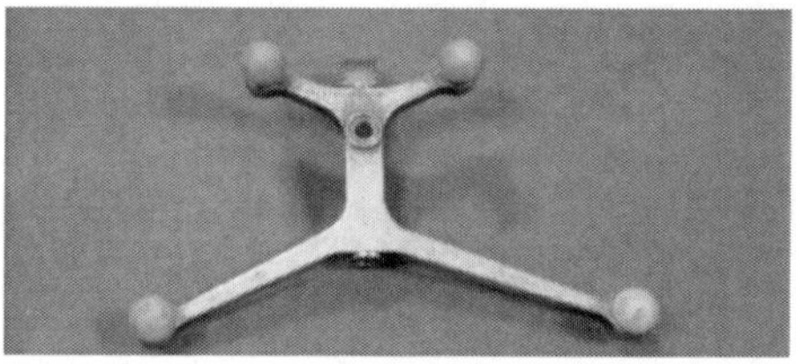

Figure 4. Dynamic reference frame (Stealthstation® Medtronic Sofamor Danek, Memphis, TN).

2.3. Procedures

Anesthesia

- General anesthesia with single lumen endotracheal tube;
- If a monitoring system for motor and somatosensory evoked potentials is required, set up prior to positional change;
- Localization of the level and entry point;
- Localization is done with portable radiograph;
- Introduction of navigation system is done after bony exposure of index level because skin incision and muscle dissection can cause anatomical deformation of skin surface. It is closely associated with accuracy of skin fixed DRF.

Cervical spine

- Mark index level with two 18-gauze needles on the skin crease of the anterior neck.

Thoracic spine

- Mark index level with 18-gauze needle and place 3-4 more needles at regular intervals to the sacral spine.

Lumbar spine

- Mark index level with 18-gauze needle
- Set up the navigation system

Cervical spine

- Supine position

While draping the patient, expose forehead widely and cover with transparent surgical film (OPSITE® Smith & Nephew, Hull, UK). Mount DRF on the skin surface of forehead and fixed firmly with incised surgical film (OPSITE® Smith & Nephew, Hull, UK) (Figure 5-7).

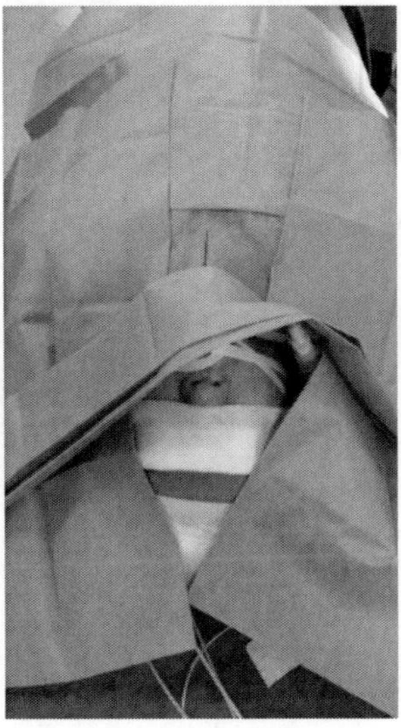

Figure 5. During the draping, expose forehead and eyes of the patient and cover eyebrows with sterile gauze to protect them from adhesive surgical film.

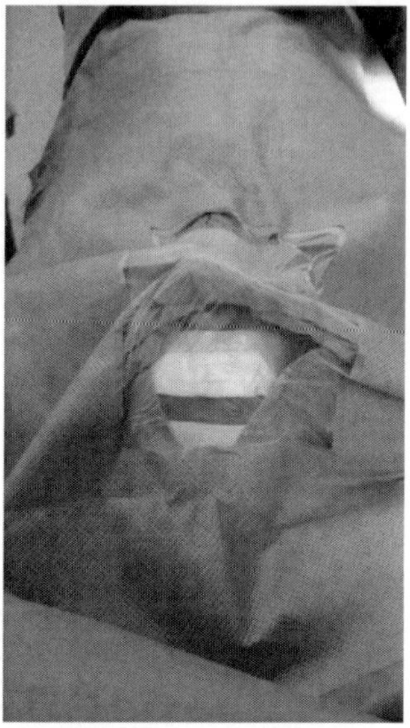

Figure 6. Exposed forehead is covered by transparent surgical film.

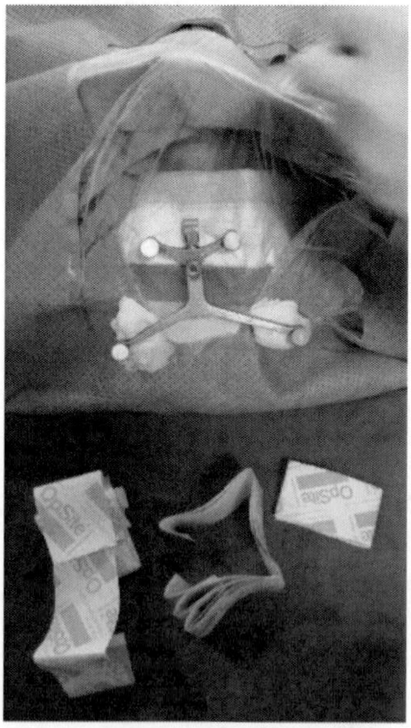

Figure 7. Mount the DRF cutaneously, overlying the draped forehead and fix it firmly with incised surgical film.

Thoracic spine

- Prone position

While draping the patient, expose the skin surface widely to the lumbar spine and cover with transparent surgical film (OPSITE® Smith & Nephew, Hull, UK). Mount DRF on the skin surface, 5-6 levels below the surgical point, and fix firmly with incised surgical film (OPSITE® Smith & Nephew, Hull, UK)

Lumbar spine

- Prone position

While draping the patient, expose the skin surface widely to the sacral hiatus area. Cover with transparent surgical film (OPSITE® Smith & Nephew, Hull, UK). Mount dynamic reference frame on the skin surface of sacral hiatus, and fix firmly with transparent surgical tape (OPSITE® Smith & Nephew, Hull, UK) (Figures 8-10).

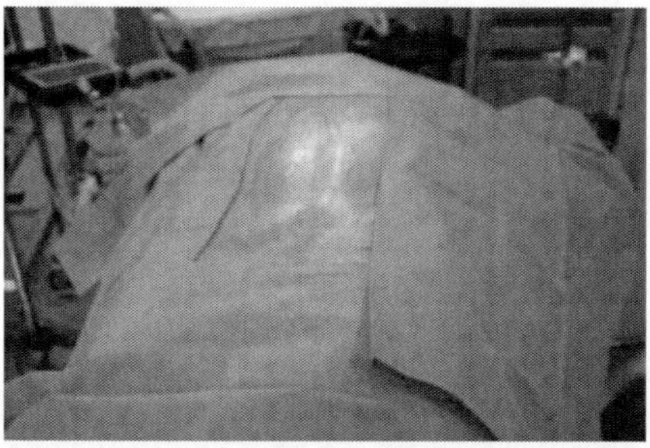

Figure 8. During the draping, expose skin surface widely to the sacral hiatus area.

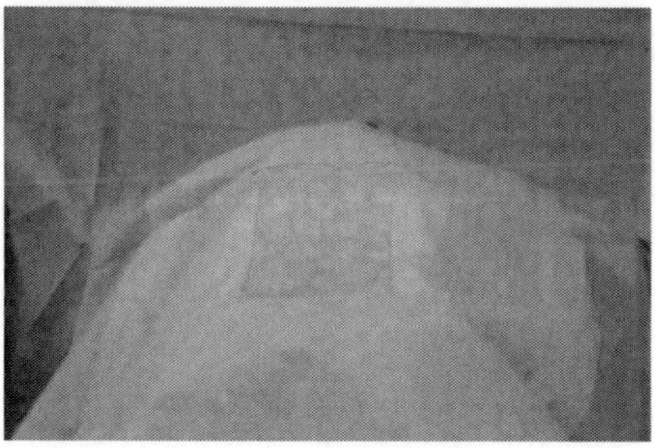

Figure 9. Exposed sacral region is covered by transparent surgical film.

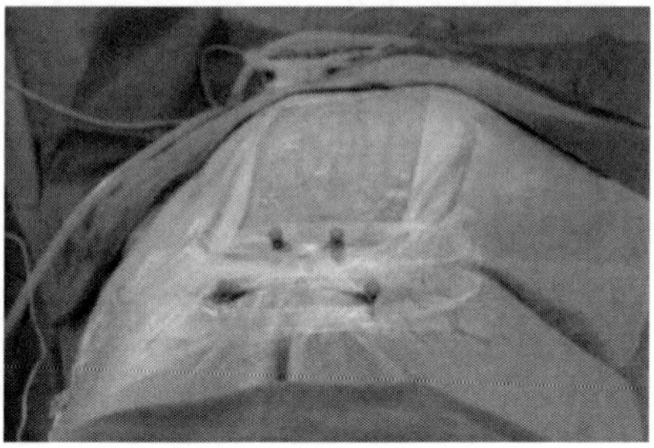

Figure 10. Mount the DRF cutaneously overlying the draped sacral hiatus area and fix it firmly with incised surgical film.

2.4. Outcomes

From June 2009 to December 2009, 20 patients underwent mini-open TLIF with skin fixed DRF [7]. Mean age was 55.9 years (range: 34–74 years) and mean BMI was 24.4 (range: 19.9–28.6).

Five patients were diagnosed with spondylolytic spondylolisthesis, and the remaining fifteen patients were diagnosed with degenerative spondylolisthesis. Nineteen patients underwent single level surgery and 1 patient underwent two-level surgery. A total of 82 screws were inserted under navigation guidance with skin fixed DRF. The mean time duration to set up the navigation system with skin fixed DRF was 8.5 ± 6.5 min (range: 10–30 min). The second O-arm scan, after pedicle screw insertion, revealed eight pedicle breaches (4 grade I, 2 grade II, and 2 grade III) [8]. Among them, the two grade III screws were reinserted and confirmed to be in the proper position with a third O-arm scan. Despite the eight pedicle perforations, there were no major complications such as nerve injury, unintended durotomy, or malposition of the final construct.

Cervical Spine

From September 2012 to May 2013, 31 patients underwent minimally invasive anterior cervical surgery. A single level surgery was done in 10 patients; two level surgeries in 11; and three level surgeries in 10. The mean time duration to set up navigation system with skin fixed DRF was 4.8 ± 3.5 min. (range: 8–20 min). 48 Caspar pins were inserted into each cervical vertebra. The validity of the navigation was then assessed by comparing the differences between the actual positions of the inserted Caspar pin, based on the second O-arm scan and the recorded images of the navigation probe. The mean horizontal error was 0.49 ± 0.71 mm. The mean vertical error was 0.88 ± 0.93 mm. And the mean angular deviation in the sagittal plane was 0.59 ± 0.55°. ICC value was 0.74 for intra-observer reliability. And there were no major complications or revision surgeries due to the navigational error. But unintended durotomy developed in 3 cases without any neural injury; all of them had severe space-occupying calcified OPLL, however, in all cases, in-situ dura repair was done with artificial dura.

CONCLUSION

With development of the navigation system, the spine surgeon can perform complex and minimal invasive surgery successfully without radiation hazard, but many surgeons are still do not favor the navigation system and don't trust it, due to the complex methods for registration and the set up process, learning curve, and the interruption of work flow. This modified method will be one part of the solution to overcome these kinds of problems.

REFERENCES

[1] Acosta, F. L., Jr., Thompson, T. L., Campbell, S., Weinstein, P. R., Ames, C. P., Use of intraoperative isocentric C-arm 3D fluoroscopy for sextant percutaneous pedicle screw placement: case report and review of the literature. *The spine journal: official journal of the North American Spine Society* 5 (3):339-343. doi:10.1016/j.spinee.2004.09.012.

[2] Fritsch, E., Duchow, J., Seil, R., Grunwald, I., Reith, W., Accuracy of fluoroscopic navigation of pedicle screws. CT-based evaluation of bone screw placement. *Der Orthopade* 31 (4):385-391, 2002.

[3] Holly, L. T., Foley, K. T., Intraoperative spinal navigation. *Spine* 28 (15 Suppl):S54-61. doi:10.1097/01.brs.0000076899.78522.d9, 2003.

[4] Tjardes, T., Shafizadeh, S., Rixen, D., Paffrath, T., Bouillon, B., Steinhausen, E. S., Baethis, H., Image-guided spine surgery: state of the art and future directions. *European spine journal: official publication of the European Spine Society, the European Spinal Deformity Society, and the European Section of the Cervical Spine Research Society* 19 (1):25-45. doi:10.1007/s00586-009-1091-9, 2010.

[5] Holly, L. T., Foley, K. T., Image guidance in spine surgery. *The Orthopedic clinics of North America* 38 (3):451-461; abstract viii. doi:10.1016/j.ocl.2007.04.001, 2007.

[6] Moses, Z. B., Mayer, R. R., Strickland, B. A., Kretzer, R. M., Wolinsky, J. P., Gokaslan, Z. L., Baaj, A. A., Neuro-navigation in minimally invasive spine surgery. *Neurosurgical focus* 35 (2):E12. doi:10.3171/2013.5.focus13150, 2013.

[7] Cho, J. Y., Chan, C. K., Lee, S. H., Lee, H. Y., The accuracy of 3D image navigation with a cutaneously fixed dynamic reference frame in minimally invasive transforaminal lumbar interbody fusion. *Computer aided surgery: official journal of the International Society for Computer Aided Surgery* 17 (6):300-309. doi:10.3109/ 10929088.2012.728625, 2012.

[8] Rajasekaran, S., Vidyadhara, S., Ramesh, P., Shetty, A. P., Randomized clinical study to compare the accuracy of navigated and non-navigated thoracic pedicle screws in deformity correction surgeries. *Spine* 32 (2):E56-64. doi:10.1097/01.brs.0000252094.64857.ab, 2007.

In: Computer-Assisted Surgery
Editor: Xiaojun Chen
ISBN: 978-1-63463-811-1

Chapter 5

ULTRASOUND IMAGING FOR ROBOTIC ORTHOPEDIC SURGERY: A SURVEY

***Pedro M. B.Torres*[*1,2] and Paulo J. S. Gonçalves[1,2]**

[1]Polytechnic Institute of Castelo Branco, School of Technology, Castelo Branco, Portugal

[2]LAETA, IDMEC, Instituto Superior Técnico, Universidade de Lisboa, Lisboa, Portugal

ABSTRACT

Robotic surgeries are performed by classical techniques, purely mechanical and their success essentially depends on the surgeon's experience. However, surgeons are increasingly receptive to new technologies and search new tools that help them improve their performance. Increasing advances in robotics have allowed the emergence of new systems dedicated to surgery, which began to be a valid option in surgical aid. The computer-assisted surgery (CAS) and particularly the robot-assisted surgery, improves accuracy and precision of procedures, allowing more reliable and reproducible outcomes, minimizing the invasiveness of surgical procedures and improving patient outcomes by reducing complications and improving patient safety compared with conventional techniques. The increasing evolution of surgical robotic systems has also been accompanied for significant evolution in surgical navigation systems.

[*] Corresponding to: Email: paulo.goncalves@ipcb.pt

Actual systems, commonly used in the operating room, employ markers placed on the human for tracking bones or other body parts. Ultrasound images are on the rise, and under strong development for use in surgeries, allowing low-cost and non-invasive real-time navigation systems.

These navigation systems will be used in the near future in CAS and robotic surgery. The chapter will review the current approaches in robotic surgery, where ultrasound based navigation is used, with a special care on orthopedics.

Keywords: Ultrasound imaging, robotics, surgical robotics

1. INTRODUCTION

Increasing advances in robotics have allowed the emergence of new systems dedicated to surgery, which began to be a valid option in surgical aid. The computer-assisted surgery (CAS) [1] and particularly the robot-assisted surgery [2, 3] improves accuracy and precision of procedures, besides producing more reliable and reproducible outcomes, minimizing the invasiveness of surgical procedures improving patient outcomes by reducing complications and improving patient safety compared with conventional orthopedic techniques.

The use of robots to automate medical tasks increases its reliability, accuracy and is an excellent contribution to Minimal Invasive Surgery (MIS). MIS is becoming more and more common nowadays in hospitals. These procedures through tiny incisions are performed instead of one large opening. Because the incisions are small, patients trend to have quicker recovery times and less discomfort than with conventional surgery. Last thirty years have been marked by the development of robotic systems for MIS. In 1985 a robot, The PUMA 560 [4] was used to place a needle for a brain biopsy using CT guidance. Three years later the same machine was used to perform a transurethral resection. In 1987 robotics was used in the first Laparoscopy surgery, a cholescystecotomy. In 1988, PROBOT, [5] developed at Imperial College London, was used to perform prostatic surgery.

More recently appeared the following surgical systems: ZEUS, DaVinci and DLR MIRO. The ZEUS robotic surgical system, initially developed in 1995 for endoscopic microsurgery (including general surgery, thoracic surgery, gynaecology, urology), was the robotic system used in the first transatlantic surgical intervention performed on a human, in 2001 between

New York and Strasbourg, France, at 15000 km of distance [6]. The DaVinci Surgical System enables surgeons to operate through a few tiny incisions with dramatically enhanced vision, precision and control. State-of-the-art DaVinci Surgery helps surgeons to minimize the pain and risk associated with traditional surgery, while increasing the chances for a fast recovery and excellent clinical outcomes.DLR MIRO [7–9] is a compact, slim and LightWeight Robot (LWR) robotic system versatile for various existing and future medical robotic procedures. It can be used in orthopedics for setting holes for bone screws, robot-assisted endoscope guidance and on to the multi-robot concept for (endoscopic) minimal invasive surgery.

2. Orthopedic Robotic Surgery

In orthopedics several solutions have emerged, such as ROBODOC® [10], for the planning and performance of total hip and knee replacement, CASPAR® [9], developed for the same purpose of ROBODOC®, Acrobot Sculptor [11, 12], used in knee surgery, or the RIO robotic arm (MAKOplasty) [13], the latest developed system for orthopedics.The Robodoc® surgical system consisted of the Orthodoc® [14], pre-surgical planner and the Robodoc® as the surgical tool. The Robodoc system comprises a five-axis Sankyo-Seiki industrial robot with a six degree-of-freedom force-sensor. The Orthodoc® describes the three-dimensional geometry of the femur from CT data and the geometry of the implant.The MAKO system consists of the well known general purpose WAM - Whole Arm Manipulator from Barrett Technology [15], for bone deburring and an optical navigation system consisting of stereo infrared cameras, and marker arrays attached to the tibia and femur. On the other hand, the Acrobot system uses their special purpose robot manipulator, while the tibia and femur are immobilized with bone clamps which are fixed through small skin incisions.

These first systems evolved with the massive usage of the computer in the operating room, as presented in the following section.

3. Computer Aided Orthopedic Surgery

The increasing evolution of surgical robotic systems has also been accompanied by significant evolution in the surgical navigation systems [16].

Of the several systems that have appeared in the market are highlighted the OrthoPilot [17], (http://www.orthopilot.com) and the BrainLAB systems [18], (https://www.brainlab.com). Both systems employ markers placed on the femur for tracking the bone movements [19].

The incisions performed to place these markers can leave serious injury to the patient and there are many cases of complaints of pain at the implant site after Surgery. Studies on the patients reported persistent severe pain at the site of pin implantation, after surgery, caused by the injuries to the nerves, caused by fiducial markers [20].

Surgical navigation systems allow the surgeon to perform surgical actions in real time using information conveyed through a virtual world, which consist of computer-generated models of surgical instruments and the virtual representations of the anatomy being operated. Virtual representations can be generated from data obtained through Computer Tomography scans, ultrasound images, amongst others. Image-guided surgical navigation is on the rise in many different areas of medicine, with strong growth in orthopedic surgery.

The use of visual information obtained from medical images is widely used in Computer Aided Orthopedic Surgery (CAOS) (www.caos-international.org). CAOS systems are increasingly available, with several commercial and research systems now well established. These systems assist surgeons in preoperative planning and simulation, from the obtained bone model, and in intra-operative navigation, using tracking systems with fiducial markers attached to the patient bone, and in the robotic execution of the surgical procedure. From the fiducial markers the position and orientation of the bone in the intra-operative scenario relative to the robot frame is obtained in the state-of-the-art systems, e.g., the Brain Lab System or Orthopilot.

Much research has been developed in order to find new solutions and explore alternatives to avoid the fiducial markers in surgical navigation, [21, 22]. The use of ultrasound (US) images has gained high relevance in Image-guided surgeries, [23, 24], since it is a non-invasive modality and provides real-time images, which are used to plan a surgical procedure and guide surgical instruments during surgery. The ultrasound based 3D bone surfaces are located by placing markers in the US probe to track them and generating a 3D bone surface that can be registered with a model preconceived through a 3D image modality, as Computed Tomography (CT) or Magnetic Resonance Imaging (MRI).

4. Towards Ultrasound Imaging in Orthopedic Surgery

Recently, much scientific research work has been developed, with the purpose of eliminating fiducial markers in orthopedic surgery [25, 26], and the main guidelines of research focuses on the use of intra-operative Ultrasound (US) images and pre-operative computed tomography (CT) to provide real time surgical guidance. In [27], it is presented a semi-automatic bone detection approach for US via registration with CT datasets pre-operatively acquired. The CT data is used to create a patient-specific bone model, and rigid transformation from US to CT is estimated by the Iterative Closest Point (ICP) algorithm, from a initializing of three points in the datasets. The three correspondence points, define the principal axis and orientation of the bone in both modalities. In [28] is proposes a point-based registration algorithm based on unscented Kalman filter (UKF) to estimate the rigid transformation parameters between the bone surfaces obtained from US and CT data, less sensitive to outliers compared with ICP.

Both methods are based on features of the datasets (feature-based), but there are also methods that use the image intensity information (intensity-based) directly in order to avoid extraction of bone surfaces. In [29] was used the normalized cross-correlation as a similarity metric for registering CT and US images. Prior to registration, both datasets were converted to bone probability images using gradient, bone intensity and US shadowing artifact information. More recently, in [30] it is proposed a rigid registration method where the translation parameters are estimated from the projections of local phase volumes in frequency domain. Bone surfaces were automatically extracted directly from 3D US and CT volumes based on 3D local image features calculated using 3D Log-Gabor filter.

After its incipient first experiments, guiding a robot using ultrasound images, i.e., ultrasound based visual servoing, has recently gained new interest due to the establishment of visual servoing.

Initial works consisted in the use of robot arms that manipulated an ultrasound probe for medical diagnoses [31, 32]. The use of ultrasound also found its way into orthopedics as a non-invasive radiation-free navigation system for surgeon operated, interventions [33]. This is particularly valuable when the bones to be operated are so small, that it is not possible to attach heavy tracking targets onto them. For interventions cooperated by robot arms, effective applications using ultrasound guidance are not yet available, but an intense race involving research centers and industry is currently taking place.

Guiding a robot in positioning tasks through visual information using uncalibrated visual servoing systems is a very active research topic due to the complexity of real applications and workspace scenarios such as an operating room. The operating room can unpredictably change during a surgery, causing calibration errors. In [34], uncalibrated visual servoing was proposed, where the inverse system Jacobean was estimated on-line, thus immune to camera miss-calibration. It presents a very promising solution for the operating room, where it is also desired to minimize calibration time. Furthermore, this approach will give added robustness to a medical setting where the environment is calibrated, but redundancy is necessary for safety reasons. This work has been further extended to a more general case in [35], where the uncalibrated model can evolve during the tasks to be performed. In [36], tools for ultrasound based 3D Bone model reconstruction; registration and visualization are presented, which are currently being developed by the research team, in order to introduce ultrasound feedback in the visual control loop. In [37], was proposed and approach to obtain the position and orientation of a bone based in it's 3D model obtained from Computed Tomography images (in the preoperative scenario) and the registration of ultrasound images to it (in the intra-operative scenario). More recently, in [38], was proposed a vision system for robotic ultrasound guided orthopedic surgery. This system, during surgery, acquires a 3D US bone surface from a sequence of US images. Later, that bone surface will then be registered to the pre-operative 3D bone model, for a precise knowledge of the bone position and orientation. The system then allows bone tracking during surgeries based on ultrasound images of bones, without the use of fiducial markers, diminishing invasiveness, is briefly presented in the next section.

5. Ultrasound Based Navigation for Orthopedic Surgery

For navigation, the system presented in [38], during surgery, acquires a 3D US bone surface from a sequence of US images. This bone surface will then be registered to the pre-operative bone model, for a precise knowledge of the bone position and orientation. This registration is performed in two steps. Firstly a global registration is performed, before the surgical procedure, to exactly register the bone. The second step is to locally register the bone, which is faster and more suitable for tracking the bone movements. To update the bone´s drilling position and orientation, the robot manipulator uses the measured bone movement. Figure 1 shows an overview of the HipRob navigation system [38].

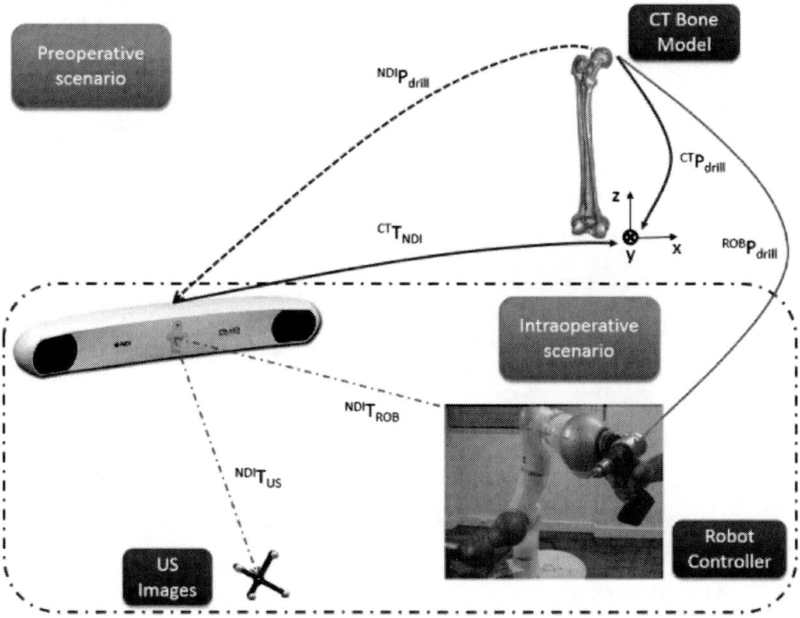

Figure 1. Overview of the hardware setup and frames transformations of HipRob navigation system [38].

The avoidance of fiducial markers implies that the US probe is referenced to the optical measurement system (NDI - Polaris) (\http://www.ndigital.com/medical/products/polaris-family). Placing on marker in the US probe makes the referencing. From this moment, also the images and features are referenced to the tracker. The pose of the robot end-effector also has to be referenced by the Navigation system to inform the robot controller of its location. The ideal drilling point is obtained pre-operatively in the CT reference frame. Inside the operating room, an initial calibration ($^{CT}T_{NDI}$) between the tracker and CT is needed to localize the femur. After calibration, the main goal consists in to determine at each instant, the drilling point in the robot reference frame ($^{ROB}P_{drill}$) and track the bone movements with the robot.

Conclusion

The present chapter presented the most important steps that surgical robotics are performing towards a common use in the operating room. The control of robots is evolving at an enormous pace and is strongly pushed by the recent advances in medical imaging. Ultrasound imaging plays a decisive role in robotic surgery because it is noninvasive and widely used by medical doctors. The main drawback is the precision of the measurements taken from US images. It was shown that this error is less than 2 [mm] nowadays, which allows its use in the operating room during surgeries. These types of systems are still slow, and cannot be operated in real-time, although they can give a measure to correct the robot trajectory. Future developments in this field will surely take care of diminishing the computational time, and also the precision of the system.

The HipRob navigation system was applied with real results in a femur phantom developed by the authors, assuring a precise calibration scheme, below 2 [mm] error, [35] which allows the ultrasound system to track the femur movements.

Acknowledgment

This work is partially supported by FCT, through IDMEC, under LAETA Pest-OE/EME/LA0022.

References

[1] Adams, L., Krybus, W., Meyer-Ebrecht, D., Rueger, R., Gilsbach, J.M., Moesges, R., Schloendorff, G., (1990). Computer-assisted surgery, *IEEE Computer Graphics and Applications*. 10(3), 43-51.

[2] Kather, J., Hagen, M.E., Morel, P., Fasel, J., Markar S, Schueler M., (2010). Robotic hip arthroscopy in human anatomy, *Int J Med Robot*. 6(3), 301-305.

[3] Mantwill, F., Schulz, A.P., Faber, A., Hollstein, D., Kammal, M., Fay, A., Ju, Ch., (2005). Robotic systems in total hip arthroplasty - is the time ripe for a new approach?, *Int J Med Robot*. 1(4), 8-19.

[4] Satava, R.M., (2002). Surgical robotics: the early chronicles: a personal historical perspective, *Surg Laparosc Endosc Percutan Tech.* 12, 6-16.

[5] Harris, S.J., Arambula-Cosio F., Mei, Q., Hibberd, R.D., Davies, B.L., Wickham, J.E., Nathan, M.S., Kundu, B. (1997). The Probot - an active robot for prostate resection, *Proc Inst Mech Eng H*, 211(4), 317-325.

[6] Marescaux, J., Leroy, J., Gagner, M., Rubino, F., Mutter, D., Vix, M., Butner, S.E., Smith, M.K., (2001). Transatlantic robot-assisted telesurgery, *Nature*, 413, 379-380.

[7] Konietschke, R., Hagn, U., Nickl, M., Jorg, S., Tobergte, A., Passig, G., Seibold, U., Le-Tien, L., Kubler, B., Groger, M., and Frohlich, F., and Rink, C., and Albu-Schaffer, A., and Grebenstein, M., and Ortmaier, T., Hirzinger, G., (2009). The DLR MiroSurge - A robotic system for surgery, *IEEE International Conference on Robotics and Automation*, 1589—1590.

[8] Hagn, U., Nickl, M., Jorg, S., Passig, G., Bahls, T., Nothhelfer, A., Hacker, F., Le-Tien, L., Albu-Schaffer, A., Konietschke, R., Grebenstein, M., Warpup, R., Haslinger, R., Frommberger, M., Hirzinger, G., (2008). The DLR MIRO: a versatile lightweight robot for surgical applications, *Industrial Robot: An International Journal*, 35(4), 324-336.

[9] Ryan, A. B., (2012). Medical Robots: Current Systems and Research Directions, *Journal of Robotics*.

[10] Kazanzides, P., Mittelstadt, B.D., Musits, B.L., Bargar, W.L., Zuhars, J.F., Williamson, B., Cain, P.W., Carbone, E.J., (1995). An integrated system for cementless hip replacement, *IEEE Engineering in Medicine and Biology Magazine*, 14(3), 307 -313.

[11] Cobb, J.P., Henckel, J., Gomes, M.P.S.F., Barrett, A.R.W., Harris, S.J., Jakopec, M., Rodriguez, F.M., Davies, B.L., (2006). Hands-on robotic unicompartmental knee replacement: a prospective, randomised controlled study of the acrobot system, *The Journal of Bone and Joint Surgery B*, 88(2), 188 -197.

[12] Davis, E.T., Gallie, P., Macgroarty, K., Waddele, J.P., Schemitsch, E., (2007). The accuracy of image-free computer navigation in the placement of the femoral component of the Birmingham Hip Resurfacing, *The Bone & Joint Journal*, 89(4), 557-560.

[13] Pearle, A. D., Kendoff, D., Stueber, V., Musahl, V., Repicci, J. A., (2009). Perioperative management of unicompartmental knee arthroplasty using the MAKO robotic arm system (MAKOplasty), *American Journal of Orthopedics*, 38(2), 16-19.

[14] Paul, H.A., Bargar, W.L., Mittlestad, B., Musits, B., Taylor, R.H., Kazanzides, P., Zuhars Willliamson, B., Hanson W., (1992). Development of a surgical robot for cementless total hip arthroplasty, *Clinical Orthopedics*, 285, 57-66.

[15] Rooks, B., (2006). The harmonious robot, *Industrial Robot: An International Journal*, 33(2), 125-130.

[16] Stiehl, J.B., Konermann, W.H., Haaker, R.G., DiGioia, A.M., (2007). Navigation and MIS in Orthopedic Surgery, *Springer.*

[17] Miehlke, R.K., Haaker, R.G., Konermann, W.H., (2004). Navigation and Robotics in Total Joint and Spine Surgery, *Navigation and Robotics in Total Joint and Spine Surgery*, 242-247.

[18] Gumprecht, H.K., Widenka, D.C., Lumenta, C.B., (1999). BrainLab VectorVision Neuronavigation System: technology and clinical experiences in 131 cases, *Neurosurgery*, 44(1), 97-104.

[19] Schulz, A.P., Faber, A., and Meiners, J., (2007). Determination of optimal non-invasive patient fixation methods for use in robotic hip replacement surgery - an in vitro study, *Int J Med Robot.* 3(2), 135--139.

[20] Nogler, M., Maurer, H., Wimmer, C., Gegenhuber, C., Bach, C., Krismer, M., (2001). Knee pain caused by a fiducial marker in the medial femoral condyle: a clinical and anatomic study of 20 cases, *Acta orthopaedica Scandinavica.* 72(5), 477-480.

[21] Barratt, D., Penney, G., Chan, C., Slomczykowski, M., Carter, T., Edwards, P., Hawkes, D., (2006). Self-calibrating 3d-ultrasound-based bone registration for minimally invasive orthopedic surgery, *IEEE Transactions on Medical Imaging*. 25(3), 312–323.

[22] Talib, H., Styner, M., Rudolph, T., Gonzalez Ballester, M., (2007). Dynamic registration using ultrasound for anatomical referencing, *4th IEEE International Symposium on Biomedical Imaging*, 1164–1167.

[23] Daanen, V., Tonetti, J., Troccaz, J., (2004). An information fusion method for the automatic delineation of the bone-soft tissues interface in ultrasound images, *Computer Vision and Mathematical Methods in Medical and Biomedical Image Analysis, LNCS*, 3117, 218–229.

[24] Hacihaliloglu, I., Abugharbieh, R., Hodgson, A., Rohling, R., (2008) Bone segmentation and fracture detection in ultrasound using 3d local phase features, *Medical Image Computing and Computer-Assisted Intervention, LNCS,* 5241, 287–295.

[25] Amiot, L., Poulin, F., (2004). Computed tomography-based navigation for hip, knee, and spine surgery, *Clin. Orthop. Relat. Res.* 421, 77-86.

[26] Nabeyama, R., Matsuda, S., Miura, H., Mawatarim, T., Kawano, T., Iwamoto, Y. (2004). The accuracy of image-guided knee replacement based on computed tomography, *Journal of Bone and Joint Surgery*. 86-B, 366-371.

[27] Beitzel, J., Ahmadi, S.A., Karamalis, A., Wein, W., Navab, N. (2012). Ultrasound bone detection using patient-specific CT prior, *International Conference of the IEEE Engineering in Medicine and Biology Society*. 2664-2667.

[28] Moghari, G.P., Barratt, D.C., Chan, C.S.K., Slomczykowski, M., Carter, T.J., Edwards, P.J., Hawkes, D.J., (2007). Point-Based Rigid-Body Registration Using an Unscented Kalman Filter, *IEEE Transactions on Medical Imaging*. 26(12), 1708-1728.

[29] Penney, M.H., Abolmaesumi, P., (2006). Cadaver validation of intensity-based ultrasound to CT registration, *Medical Image Analysis*. 10(3), 385-395.

[30] Hacihaliloglu, I., Wilson, D.R.. Gilbart, M., Hunt, M.A., Abolmaesumi, P., (2013). Non-iterative partial view 3D ultrasound to CT registration in ultrasound-guided computer-assisted orthopedic surgery, *International Journal of Computer Assisted Radiology and Surgery*. 8(2), 157-168.

[31] Abolmaesumi, P., Salcudean, S.E., Wen-Hong Z., Sirouspour, M.R., DiMaio, S.P., (2002). Image-guided control of a robot for medical ultrasound, *IEEE Transactions on Robotics and Automation*. 18(1), 11-23.

[32] Krupa, A., Chaumette, F., (2006). Guidance of an ultrasound probe by visual servoing, *Advanced Robotics*. 20(11), 1203-1218.

[33] Chen, T., Abolmaesumi, P., Pichora, D.R., Ellis, R.E., (2005). A System for Ultrasoundguided Computer-assisted Orthopaedic Surgery, *Journal of Computer Aided Surgery*. 10(5-6), 281-292.

[34] Goncalves, P.J.S., Mendonca, L.F., Sousa, J.M.C., Caldas Pinto, J.R., (2008). Uncalibrated Eye-to-Hand Visual Servoing using Inverse Fuzzy Models, *IEEE Transactions on Fuzzy Systems*. 16(2), 341-353.

[35] Goncalves, P.J.S., Sousa, J.M.C., Caldas Pinto, J.R., (2008). Evolving Fuzzy Modeling of an Uncalibrated Visual Servoing System, *In Lecture Notes in Computer Science, Springer-Verlag Berlin*. 5112, 1041-1050.

[36] Goncalves, P.J.S., Fernandes, J.M., (2008). Tools for an Ultrasound Based 3D Bone Model Reconstruction, Registration and Visualization System, *Euromedia 2008, Workshop on Medical Imaging Systens, Porto, Portugal*.

[37] Goncalves, P.J.S., Carvalho, M. V., Mateus, D., Torres P.M.B., (2009). Registo de Imagens Ecográficas com Modelo 3D de Ossos - aplicação ao fémur, *Revista Ibérica de Sistemas e Tecnologias de Informação*. 4, 43-56.

[38] Gonçalves, P.J.S., Torres, P.M.B., Santos, F. and António, R., Catarino, N., Martins, J.M.M., (2014). A Vision System for Robotic Ultrasound Guided Orthopedic Surgery, *Journal of Intelligent & Robotic Systems*. 1-13.

In: Computer-Assisted Surgery
Editor: Xiaojun Chen
ISBN: 978-1-63463-811-1

Chapter 6

DEVELOPMENT OF SCRUB NURSE ROBOT (SNR) SYSTEMS FOR LAPAROSCOPIC SURGERY

Kitaro Yoshimitsu [*]
Institute of Advanced Biomedical Engineering and Science (TWIns),
Faculty of Advanced Techno-Surgery (FATS),
Tokyo Women's Medical University, Japan

ABSTRACT

There is currently a chronic shortage of scrub nurses to exchange surgical instruments with operating surgeons. Smooth instrument exchange maintains a surgeon's operating rhythm and can be limited by the availability of skilled scrub nurses. To compensate for this shortage, we propose a scrub nurse robot (SNR), which will achieve an efficacy at the level of a skilled human scrub nurse during laparoscopic surgery. In this paper, we developed a new SNR with a novel function: automatic insertion of a surgical instrument to achieve a smooth instrument exchange with the expectation that the higher functional ability would increase surgical operation efficacy. First, we developed the first version of the SNR, which was composed of two separate robots called R-1and R-2. The R-1 was designed to have two arms to handle an electric knife

[*] Correspondence to: 8-1 Kawada-cho, Shinjuku-ku, Tokyo, 162-8666, Japan. Email: yoshimitsu. kitaro@twmu.ac.jp.

and a blood aspirator, which are the instruments that are most frequently used during laparoscopic surgery. The R-2 has a horizontal arm and two hands. The R-2 also has a tool changer that stores other instruments. After the basic validation study of the first SNR, the second version of the SNR was developed and achieved smooth and wide movement of its arms, each with four degrees of freedom (DOF). The second SNR is able to speak several sentences and recognize some words, as well as the names of surgical instruments, and is also capable of recognizing a surgeon's intraoperative actions by a real-time visual recognition system (RTVRS). The RTVRS is basically composed of both a commercially available three-dimensional (3D) position-tracking system and the algorithm that we developed to recognize the surgeon's actions during the exchange of instruments from the aforementioned positional data. Considering the results from the validation study of the second SNR, the third version of the SNR, which is able to insert the tip of the instrument into a small-caliber trocar cannula penetrating a patient's abdominal wall, was developed. This function is called the automatic instrument inserting function (AIIF). The AIIF's algorithm, which is called kinematic-based feedback control, enables the arm instead of a surgeon to insert the instrument into the cannula. We validated that it was quicker to use the third SNR to help the surgeon's stand-ins to exchange instruments in a laboratory using the second SNR compared to human scrub nurses in real surgical operations. We defined the time spent exchanging surgical instruments as the *targeting time*. The results of the evaluation showed that it was possible to exchange instruments 1.69 s faster than in a clinical operating room between a human scrub nurse and a surgeon and 2.8 s faster than using the second SNR.

Keywords: Laparoscopic surgery, robotic scrub nurse, automatic instrument inserting function

1. Introduction

Large hospitals continue to face a chronic shortage of nurses. The shortage is especially dire for scrub nurses who assist surgeons by exchanging surgical instruments [1, 2]. A scrub nurse is required to hand a surgical instrument to an operating surgeon as soon as it is requested. It may cause a distraction during the overall procedure if the scrub nurse spends too much time looking for the instrument. This lag may place an unnecessary burden on the surgeon, possibly reducing the quality and efficacy of the operation. To avoid such delays, the scrub nurse needs to be fully attentive to the activity in the operative field and also accurately anticipate what instrument a surgeon might need in the next procedure. For this to be possible, the scrub nurse needs to know the surgical procedure and the surgeon and also must be highly disciplined. An ideal scrub nurse is defined as someone who is able to meet the aforementioned requirements; as such, ideal scrub nurses are scarce. To compensate for the severe shortage of scrub nurses, a scrub nurse robot (SNR) system has been proposed. The goal of this research project was to develop an SNR capable of acting like the aforementioned skilled scrub nurse. The SNR was designed to adapt to surgeons with various levels of skill and different personalities. Three versions of SNR systems have already developed for endoscopic and laparoscopic surgery. The target for this SNR system is laparoscopic surgery because it is not too complicated for the SNR to follow, and surgeons performing endoscopic and laparoscopic surgery do not use as many types of surgical instruments as in conventional surgery in which the abdominal or thoracic wall is cut open widely [3].

Robotic scrub nurses to pass surgical instruments have been extensively proposed and investigated. The Penelope Surgical Instrument Server (SIS) is a robotic scrub nurse that has been used in clinical cases [4]. It can hand surgical instruments to surgeons per voice commands. This robot seems to be designed for so-called minor surgeries. Takashima et al. [5] have developed an interface between their own developed robotic scrub nurse and a surgeon, although the system has not yet been used in actual clinical cases. However, the SNR system that is proposed herein is intended to be used during major surgery such as abdominal, thoracic, and cardiac surgery. Moreover, the goals of the SNR are for it to be able to accurately anticipate which instrument the surgeon will request for the next step of surgery and to hand this to the surgeon in a timely fashion.

2. Methods

2.1. First Version of SNR

Figure 1 shows the first version of the SNR: R-1 and R-2 [6, 7].

The specifications of the R-1 (Figure 1a) were determined from analysis of the intraoperative motions of a surgeon and a scrub nurse in laparoscopic surgery [2]. In the preliminary investigation of a laparoscopic cholecystectomy, an electric knife and a blood aspirator were used very frequently (for approximately 40–50% of the duration of the laparoscopic procedure). The analysis of the intraoperative motion data indicated the necessity for the robot, which handles only an electric knife and a blood aspirator, and it was decided to divide the required tasks into two robots. The R-2 (Figure 1b) was designed to handle other instruments. The total number of instruments was, at the most, 15 in a routine laparoscopic cholecystectomy. Further details about the R-1 and R-2 are described in the next chapter.

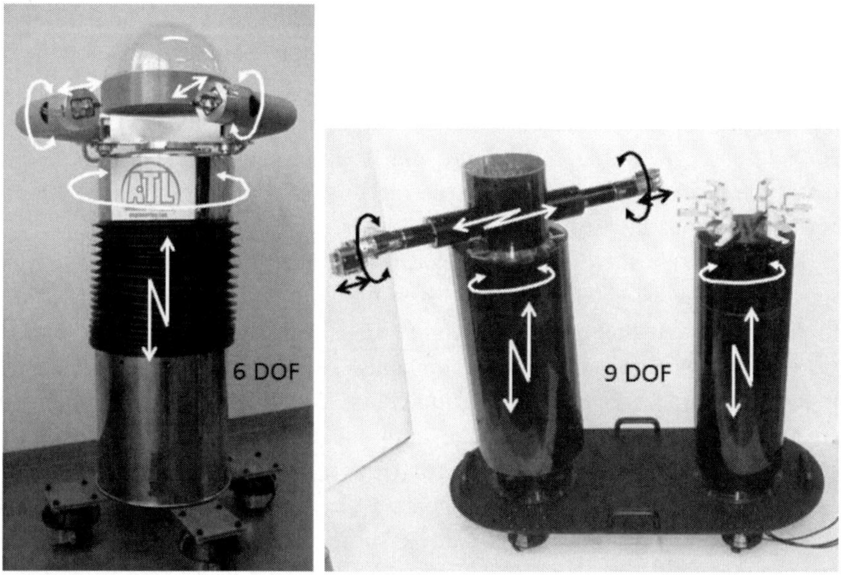

Figure 1. The first version of the SNR: R-1 and R-2.

The R-1 has a linear actuator inside its main body to lift the arm up and down to the height position of the surgeon's hand. A rotary actuator is located on this linear actuator to move the shoulders. In the wrist section, in order to realize a smooth transfer of instruments, a rotary actuator is fitted for each wrist. In the fingers, pneumatic robotic hand actuators are used to tightly grasp instruments. The R-1 has six degrees of freedom (DOF). Motor drivers and power supplies that control the actuators are located in the head section.

Figure 1b shows the R-2. The R-2 has a tool changer component and an arm component side by side. The tool changer holds a laparoscope, forceps, and the other instruments, and the arm component hands over and receives the instruments with its two hands. The tool changer has a pneumatic latch rotor actuator to transfer the instruments to the hand. The arm turns 180 degrees to pass them to the surgeon after retrieving the instrument from the tool changer. The fingers of the R-2 are moved by the same air-powered mechanism as that of the R-1 to tightly grasp instruments. The tool changer and arm components both have linear actuators for height adjustment according to the hand position of the surgeon. The R-2 has nine DOF.

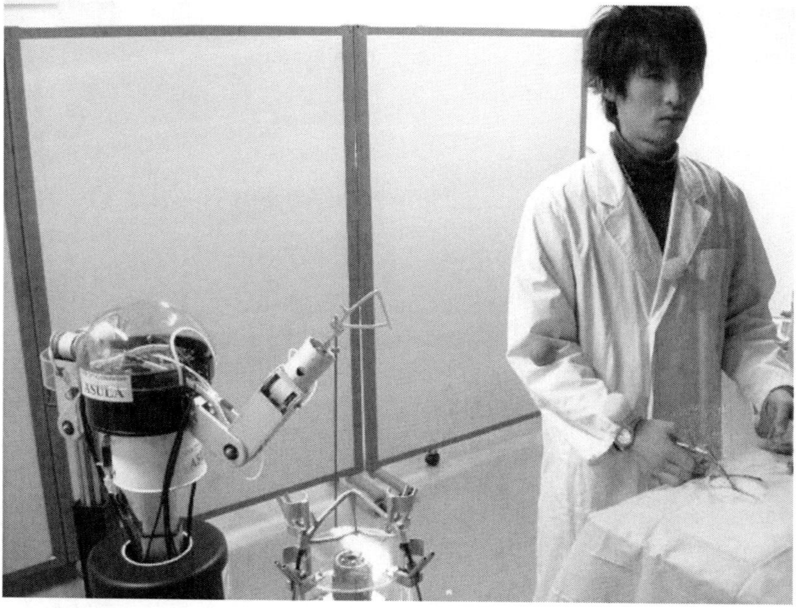

Figure 2. The second version of the SNR: ASULA.

2.2. Second Version Of SNR

Considering the results from the validation study, a second version of the SNR—termed the advanced surgical unit in laparoscopic area (ASULA)—was developed. Figure 2 shows the ASULA. The biggest change from the first version of the SNR was that the separate robots were combined into one ASULA because the first SNR was too large for ordinary operating rooms. Therefore, the working space for an SNR in an operating room is expected to be decreased, and the dangers of interference with other surgical systems and instruments could be reduced. In order to abandon the R-2's main component of the tool changer—a surgical tray, which generally holds sterilized surgical instruments—was located at the side of the ASULA. The number of DOF in the arm sections was increased to four. While the arms were now freer, use of the rotary and linear actuators was maintained. Therefore, in the second version of the SNR, a reduction by five DOF from the first version of the SNR was incorporated to offer a total of 10 DOFs. This means that even if by any chance a malfunction should occur in the SNR, safety would be improved because of the expected greater simplicity of the control program. As for the user interface, in addition to foot switches that were already installed in the first version of the SNR, a speech recognition system (Voice Key ver. 1.4) was employed to improve human adaptation.

2.3. Real-time Visual Recognition System For Second Version of SNR

We intended to develop an SNR that was capable of providing the correct instrument without any verbal requests from the surgeon and without any delay. For this to be possible, the SNR needed a real-time visual recognition system (RTVRS) to detect the characteristics of surgeons' motions when exchanging instruments, especially to detect the moment when they draw out an instrument after use.

First, we defined and divided the intraoperative actions of a surgeon into two groups: *working* and *exchanging* actions. The *working* action means that a surgeon is doing some kind of surgical procedure with a surgical instrument, and the *exchanging* action means that he or she is replacing the surgical instrument after use with the instrument that is needed next. During this exchanging action, a scrub nurse must help the surgeon in an accurate and timely manner. The exchanging action was, for the purpose of convenience, further subdivided into five key actions: (1) pulling an instrument after use through a trocar cannula; (2) returning the instrument; (3) waiting for an instrument that the surgeon has requested; (4) receiving it; and (5) inserting it into the trocar cannula.

An algorithm capable of detecting and distinguishing the surgeon's motions observed during the action of exchanging instruments was developed [8, 9]. Reflective markers were attached to the surgeon's wrist, elbow, shoulder, and chest. These markers were captured by two digital video cameras set up in the operating room. We verified whether the algorithm was capable of detecting and distinguishing the six motions observed during the aforementioned five actions. As a result, the algorithm correctly captured each motion in real surgical operations [8, 9]. The entire procedural model of an endoscopic and laparoscopic surgery was constructed for the actions of a surgeon, a scrub nurse, and the possible statuses of a patient [2, 8, 9, 10] using the extended timed-automata formalism of UPPAAL [11, 12]. This surgical model installed into the SNR can enable the SNR to know which procedure is occurring to confirm which action a surgeon is now conducting and possibly to recognize what type of surgery is happening. The aforementioned surgeon's actions can be constructed by extended timed-automata modeling, as shown in Figure 3.

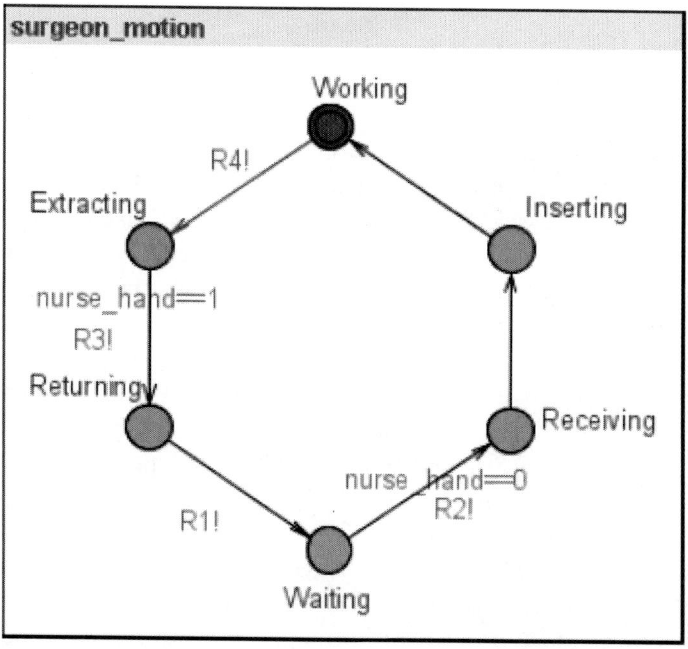

Figure 3. The aforementioned surgeon's actions during laparoscopic surgical procedure.

The composition of the first version of the RTVRS for the SNR was aimed at detecting surgeons' motions during the exchange of instruments, although the goal for the RTVRS for the SNR is to establish a visual system that enables the SNR to recognize surgical personnel actions and surgical instruments' positions in real time. First, in order to obtain real-time positional data of a surgeon's body parts, a commercially available real-time three-dimensional (3D) position-tracking system was utilized. This consists of high-speed digital video cameras with a sampling rate of 60 frames/s and QuickMag

IV, which is capable of automatically tracking colored markers and outputting their 3D coordinates. More than two digital video cameras must be used in order to provide 3D positional data. Second, we modified the aforementioned algorithm for offline analysis of a surgeon's motions in order for the SNR to recognize the surgeon's actions in real time from the 3D positional data output by the QuickMag IV. One of the main modifications was that the modified algorithm detected only two out of the six actions shown in Figure 3: extracting and inserting [13].

2.4. Third Version of SNR

Precise analysis during endoscopic and laparoscopic surgery provided us with various types of intraoperative information and findings. For example, the exchange of surgical instruments is repeated 60 to 150 times in a single laparoscopic cholecystectomy, and each action of exchanging surgical instruments takes quite a long time—on average, 4–5 s. As mentioned in the previous section, we further investigated the surgeon's actions of exchanging instruments by dividing these into five subactions, such as extracting an instrument, returning it, waiting for the next instrument, getting it from a scrub nurse, and inserting it through a trocar cannula into the operative field. We found that an older, more highly skilled surgeon spent more time inserting a surgical instrument into an inlet of a small-caliber trocar cannula than a younger novice surgeon did, although he finished the surgical operation much more quickly [7]. The action of inserting instruments into small-caliber trocar cannulas can be stressful for older surgeons because they must repeat this action many times. This action can also be unfavorable for young surgeons, although they are able to finish this action in shorter periods of time because they repeat this action many more times—sometimes amounting to 150 times in a single operation—than older, more highly skilled surgeons. Then, we came up with an idea for a new function of the SNR: an automatic instrument inserting function (AIIF). Namely, we considered that the SNR would be extremely helpful for all surgeons if the SNR instead of surgeons could insert surgical instruments into trocar cannulas. We also noticed another unfavorable action during endoscopic and laparoscopic surgery. The action of exchanging surgical instruments forces surgeons to shift their eyes from the endoscope monitor displaying the operative field. This action—called *eye-off* action—is distracting to surgeons because they like to keep their attention on the operative field. This aforementioned new feature of the SNR may eliminate this unfavorable action because surgeons will not need to look at the inlet of the trocar cannula.

According to the concept of the new feature, we developed the third version of the SNR (Figure 4). The SNR is composed of three parts: an arm, a tool changer, and a body. The arm handles an instrument and guides the tip to the entry point of a cannula. The tool changer locates the upper part of the body with the tool stage. Each holder on the tool stage grasps a surgical instrument. The body contains a power supply, electric air valves, and motor drivers in a control box at the bottom of the body.

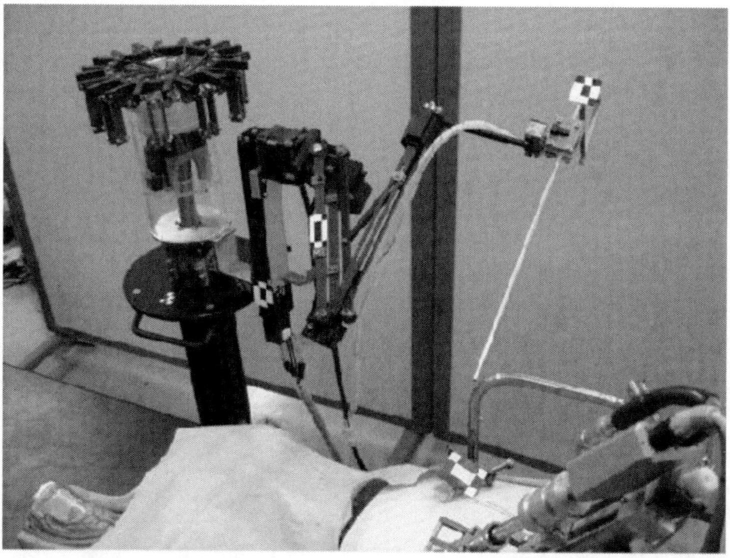

Figure 4. The third version of the SNR.

The entire arm can be detached at the shoulder by sliding respective counterparts in or out that are mutually complementary in shape. Two pneumatic actuators are used on the detachable section instead of an electric actuator in order to be sterilized. One of the actuators has two fingers and is used with a hand part to grasp an instrument with a 10-mm stroke. An infrared sensor is located on this actuator to detect objects between the fingers. The other pneumatic actuator is located at the wrist part. This actuator is used to retrieve an instrument from the tool changer. Electric drive actuators are used for the reaching mechanism, and a rotating mechanism is located at the shoulder. The shoulder rotation is correctly transmitted by using concavo-convex parts. The main shafts of the arm are made of carbon materials that are rigid and light. Every joint is made of an aluminum alloy with a black alumite treatment to prevent corrosion. Shafts in the joints are made of stainless steel with oil-less bearings. The tool changer has 10 tool holders that are positioned circularly, facing outward. This holder is designed to be detachable, similar to the arm. Each holder is composed of a pneumatic actuator and an infrared sensor to detect an instrument that is returned between the fingers. Stainless steel plates are affixed to the tip of the actuator to tightly hold an instrument. The tool stage on the tool changer is made of white MC nylon. Air pressure and electric supply for the pneumatic actuators are supplied from the control box at the bottom. At the connecting part between the tool stage and the tool changer, we used air and electric connectors to transfer air pressure and electric signals. Thus, the tool stage can also be easily detached, much like the arm.

2.5. AIIF

The greatest characteristic of the third SNR is the AIIF of its arm. The arm inserts the tip of an instrument into the entrance of the trocar cannula instead of a surgeon. The AIIF has two purposes. One of these is reducing the waiting time; this forces a surgeon to wait for the next instrument until a scrub nurse hands it to him or her—1.71 s on average. The other purpose is decreasing the eye-off time, which takes 1.41 s on average when a surgeon inserts an instrument into the trocar cannula. Inserting an instrument with a length of approximately 400 mm into a 5-mm-diameter trocar cannula can be a difficult task, especially for older surgeons. If this annoying task were done automatically by the SNR, the operating procedure would be expected to become much smoother. To achieve this feature, a 3D coordinate measurement system named Micron Tracker 2 (Claron Technology Inc.) was used as the position feedback sensor. This system obtains the 3D coordinate and angle values of specific predefined markers. In this paper, we propose kinematic-based feedback control as a controlling algorithm for the AIIF. To achieve this idea, the original position of the SNR coordinate system was set as an absolute coordinate system; reference vectors were also created, as shown in Figure 5.

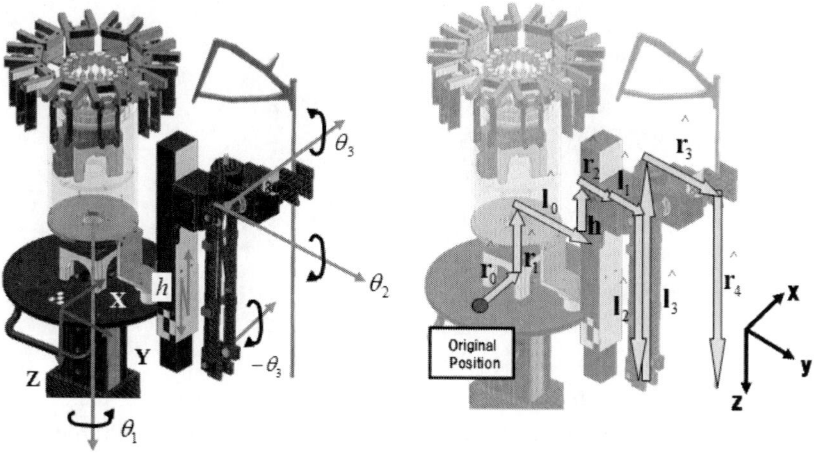

Figure 5. A controlling algorithm for the AIIF.

The AIIF was executed as follows:

- First, for the direct kinematic analysis, we described the 3D position of the tip of the instrument, as shown in Equation (1).
- Second, the 3D position of the tip of an instrument and the entrance of the trocar cannula were fed back by the Micron Tracker 2 and assigned to P_x, P_y, and P_z and P_x', P_y', and P_z', respectively.
- Third, Equation (1) was solved for simultaneously. To solve the simultaneous equations, the value of was fixed as 45 degrees.
- Finally, the values that should be controlled by each actuator were calculated via Equations (2)–(4) by using the solutions of Equation (1).

$$\begin{cases} (P_x, P_x') = \mathbf{r}_0 - S_1(\mathbf{l}_0 + \mathbf{r}_2) + (S_1S_3 + S_2C_1C_3)\mathbf{l}_2 - S_1\mathbf{r}_3 + S_2C_1(\mathbf{r}_4 - \mathbf{l}_3) \\ (P_y, P_y') = C_1(\mathbf{l}_0 + \mathbf{r}_2) + (-S_3C_1 + S_1S_2C_3)\mathbf{l}_2 + C_1\mathbf{r}_3 + S_1S_2(\mathbf{r}_4 - \mathbf{l}_3) \\ (P_z, P_z') = -\mathbf{r}_1 - \mathbf{h} + C_2C_3\mathbf{l}_2 + C_2(\mathbf{r}_4 - \mathbf{l}_3) \end{cases} \tag{1}$$

$$\theta_1 = {}^{SNRbody}_{Cannula}\theta_1{}' - {}^{SNRbody}_{Tooltip}\theta_1 \tag{2}$$

$$\theta_3 = {}^{SNRbody}_{Cannula}\theta_3' - {}^{SNRbody}_{Tooltip}\theta_3 \quad (3)$$

$$h = {}^{SNRbody}_{Cannula}h' - {}^{SNRbody}_{Tooltip}h \quad (4)$$

2.6. Evaluation of Third SNR Compared with Previous Version

In this section, we tested how fast the SNR inserts the tip of an instrument into the entrance of the trocar cannula. Four students were used as the surgeon's stand-ins in this experiment. They were all familiar with the role of a surgeon. We measured the time that was taken for the AIIF and defined this time as the *targeting time*. This targeting time starts from the moment when the tip of instrument is extracted from the entrance of the cannula. Measurement is finished at the moment when the tip of the next instrument is inserted into the cannula.

The SNR started moving from its waiting position. The signal from the infrared sensor was the trigger signal for starting the AIIF. After insertion, the surgeon's stand-ins could recognize the end of the targeting motion from a beeping sound from the computer. Then, they pushed the foot switch next to their feet. Finally, the SNR released the instrument and moved back to its original position, ready for the next motion.

The results are shown in Table I; Figure 6 shows the time taken for each segmented action. We segmented these actions based on the following definitions:

Returning: The moment from when the tip of the instrument is extracted to the moment when the surgeon releases the instrument.

Waiting: The moment from when the surgeon releases the instrument that he or she has finished using to the moment when the surgeon receives the instrument that he or she requested for the next operating procedure.

Targeting at the entrance of the cannula: The moment from when the surgeon receives the instrument that he or she will use in the next operating procedure to the moment when the surgeon inserts the tip of the instrument into the entrance of the cannula.

Mechanical movement: The moment from when the infrared sensor recognizes the extraction and the SNR starts moving to the moment when the SNR inserts the tip of the instrument into the entrance of the cannula.

Table 1. Time for targeting an instrument (in seconds)

Average	±Standard deviation	Maximum	Minimum
Surgeon: real nurses (*N* = 128)	3.72 ± 2.19	17.70	1.77
Stand-ins: second SNR (*N* = 27)	4.80 ± 0.90	6.60	2.93
Stand-ins : third SNR (*N* = 20) (Kinematic-based feedback control)	2.03 ± 0.10	2.24	1.86

The targeting time in the case of the laboratory was considerably shorter and more stable than in the case when the second SNR was used, even compared to real operations. In particular, we determined that the third SNR finished its targeting motion 1.69 s faster than clinical cases under kinematic-based feedback control. We also observed that three-fourths of the stand-ins quickly adjusted to exchanging instruments with the SNR. Afterward, most of the time, they had already or concurrently grasped the handle of the instrument when the AIIF finished. Thus, all they had to do was quickly slide in the instrument as soon as the AIIF had finished. Therefore, if this arm is introduced in clinical operating rooms, we can expect that surgeons would concentrate more on the operating procedures because the SNR would enable them not to have to pay attention to confirming the position of the entrance of the trocar cannula as surgeons do currently.

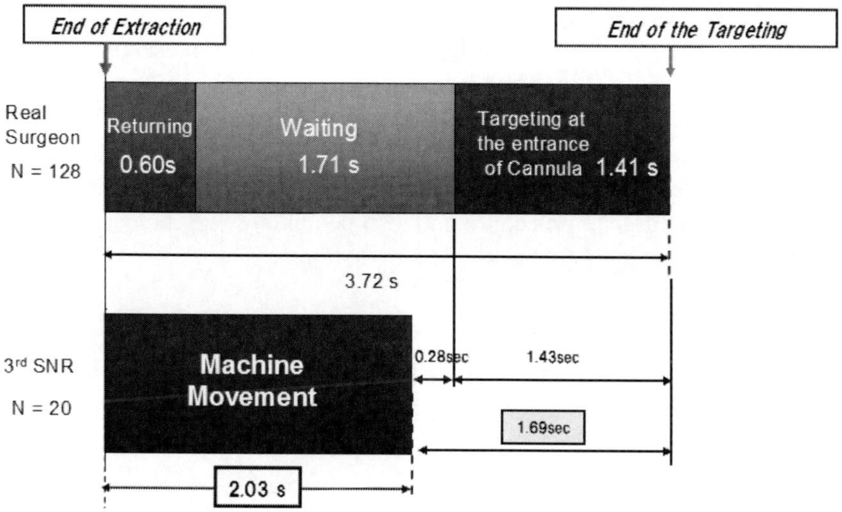

Figure 6. The time taken for each segmented action.

Conclusion

To compensate for the severe and chronic shortage of scrub nurses, we have proposed an SNR system that is capable of functioning as a skilled human scrub nurse in endoscopic and laparoscopic surgery. We have proposed and developed three versions of this system. In this paper, we describe these three versions of the SNR and its features. The first SNR, which was composed of two separate robots called R-1 and R-2, was designed as a prototype. After the basic evaluation of the first SNR, we developed the second version of the SNR, which has a voice recognition system as a user interface and achieved smooth and wide movement of its arms, each with four DOF. The second SNR was able to speak several sentences and recognize some words, as well as the names of surgical instruments, and was also capable of recognizing a surgeon's intraoperative actions by its RTVRS. Concerning the results from the evaluation of the second SNR, we developed the third version of the SNR, which has an AIIF. This function (instead of a surgeon) correctly inserts the next instrument into the cannula. We constructed two types of algorithms for AIIF control and evaluated how well the third SNR worked in a laboratory compared to human scrub nurses in real operations and compared to the second SNR. We discovered two remarkable results from the third SNR. One is the targeting time, which is defined as the moment from the end of extraction to the insertion of the next instrument. The third SNR was 1.69 s faster than human scrub nurses in presenting surgical instruments under the kinematic-based feedback control. Currently, we are researching how to control the SNR based on the surgical operating model that we have constructed with UPPAAL [8, 12]. By including this surgical model in the SNR system, it will be able to predict the next instrument that should be used in the next surgical procedure and also be able to work better to provide the best support for high-quality surgical operations.

References

[1] Bower, F. L., and McCullough, C., Nurse shortage or nursing shortage: Have we missed the real problem? *Nurs. Econ.*, 22(4):200-203, 2004.

[2] Miyawaki, F., Masamune, K., Suzuki, S., Yoshimitsu, K., and Vain, J., Scrub nurse robot system—Intraoperative motion analysis of a scrub

nurse and timed-automata-based model for surgery. *IEEE Trans. Ind. Electron.,* 52(5):1227-1235, 2005.

[3] Hashimoto, D., Advanced Techniques in Gasless Laparoscopic Surgery, 1995.

[4] Robotic Surgical Tech, Inc., http://www.roboticsurgicaltech.com/index.html.

[5] Takashima, K., Nakashima, H., Mukai, T., and Hayashi, S., Scrub nurse robot for laparoscopic surgery. *Adv. Robotics,* 22(13-14):1585-1601, 2008.

[6] Yoshimitsu, K., Tanaka, T., Ohnuma, K., Miyawaki, F., Hashimoto, D., and Masamune, K., Prototype development of scrub nurse robot for laparoscopic surgery, *Proceedings of Computer Assisted Radiology and Surgery*, 845-850, 2005.

[7] Yoshimitsu, K., Masamune, K., Tanaka, T., Ohnuma, K., Hashimoto, D., and Miyawaki F., Development of human adaptive scrub nurse robot for laparoscopic surgery, *Proceedings of the 3rd COE Workshop on Human Adaptive Mechatronics (HAM)*, 149-152, 2006.

[8] Ohnuma, K., Masamune, K., Yoshimitsu, K., Vain, J., Fukui, Y., and Miyawaki, F., Analysis and recognition of a surgeon's motions in laparoscopic cholecystectomy giving a scrub nurse robot suitable timings for instrument exchange, *Proceedings of the 3rd COE Workshop on Human Adaptive Mechatronics (HAM)*, 219-223, 2006.

[9] Ohnuma, K., Masamune, K., Yoshimitsu, K., Sadahiro, T., Vain, J., Fukui, Y., and Miyawaki, F., Timed-automata based model for laparoscopic surgery and intraoperative motion recognition of a surgeon as the interface connecting the surgical scenario and the real operating room, *Proceedings of Computer Assisted Radiology and Surgery*, 1(Suppl. 1):442-445, 2006.

[10] Miyawaki, F., Masamune, K., Suzuki, S., Yoshimitsu, K., and Vain, J., Intraoperative motion analysis of surgical staff and timed automata based model of surgery to develop scrub nurse robot system, *Proceedings of the 2nd COE Workshop on Human Adaptive Mechatronics (HAM)*, 65-70, 2005.

[11] Hune, T., Larsen, K., and Pettersson, P., Guided synthesis of control programs using UPPAAL, *Proceedings of the IEEE ICDCS International Workshop on Distributed Systems Verification and Validation*, E15-E22, 2000. Wang, J., Fundamentals of erbium-doped fiber amplifiers arrays, *IEEE J. Quantum Electron.*, submitted for publication.

[12] http:// www.uppaal.com.
[13] Miyawaki, F., Ohnuma, K., Sadahiro, T., Yoshimitsu, K., Masamune, K., and Fukui, Y., Development of real-time visual recognition system (RTVRS) for SNR and assessment of performance of RTVRS-driven SNR during exchange of surgical instruments, *Proceedings of the 4th COE Workshop on Human Adaptive Mechatronics (HAM)*, 25-30, 2007.

In: Computer-Assisted Surgery
Editor: Xiaojun Chen
ISBN: 978-1-63463-811-1

Chapter 7

T-CELL SHAPE VARIATION WITH INTRA-CELLULAR CA^{2+} CONCENTRATION: A JOINT IMAGE AND SHAPE STUDY

Yi Gao[1,*], ***Wei Chen***[2,3], ***Baoyu Liu***[2], ***Allen Tannenbaum***[4] ***and Cheng Zhu***[2]
[1]Stony Brook University, Dept. Biomedical Informatics, Stony Brook, NY, US
[2]Georgia Institute of Technology, Dept. Biomedical Engineering, Atlanta, GA, US
[3]School of Medicine, Zhejiang University, Hangzhou, China
[4]Stony Brook University, Depts. Computer Science and Applied Mathematics/Statistics, Stony Brook, NY, US

Abstract

Ca^{2+} signaling is of major importance for a wide range of intra- and inter-cellular processes. In particular, for the immune system, Ca^{2+} regulation is crucial for mast cell degranulation, lysis of infected cells, and essentially all responses initiated by T-cell, B-cell, and Fc receptors. The introduction of the Ca^{2+} indicators, such as the fura-2 and indo-1, by Roger Tsien and collaborators, enables the in-vivo and real time imaging of the intracellular Ca^{2+} concentration. In this work, we utilize active

*E-mail address: gaoyi@gatech.edu

contour and optimal mass transport techniques to collectively estimate the intracellular Ca^{2+} concentration and quantify the shape variations in the T-cells. Our results indicate an potentially interesting positive correlation between the intracellular Ca^{2+} concentration with the variations in T-cell shape.

1. Introduction

Ca^{2+} signaling is crucial for a wide range of intra- and inter-cellular processes including those of the immune system. Indeed, Ca^{2+} regulation is central for mast cell degranulation, lysis of infected cells, and just about all responses initiated by T-cell, B-cell, and Fc receptors [1]. Since the 1980s, the introduction of the Ca^{2+} indicators such as the fura-2 and indo-1 by Roger Tsien and collaborators [2], enables the in-vivo and real time measurement of the intracellular Ca^{2+} concentration. As a result, researchers are now able to capture the fluorescent images as well as videos, and quantitatively estimate the dynamics of intracellular Ca^{2+} concentration.

In this note, we utilize the 340nm/380nm two channel fluorescent images by collectively analyzing the Ca^{2+} concentration as well as the variation of the shape of the T-cell. Using the active contour method [3], we automatically identify and track the T-cell within the high-speed camera video. After that, based on the optimal mass transport theory [4], we formulate a metric to quantify the "distance" between cell shape configurations. The resulting time-varying Ca^{2+} concentration and the shape metric curves shows an interesting positive correlation, which may provide insight into the study of immunological function of the T-cell.

2. Method

In this section, we first describe how to extract and segment a given cell from the 380nm fluorescent image. Then, based on the segmentation, we estimate the Ca^{2+} concentration and the shape change in the cell, and determine the correlation between them.

2.1. Cell Extraction and Tracking

In order to estimate the intra cellular Ca^{2+} concentration as well as to compute the shape of the cell, we have to extract the boundary of the cell from the video. To that end, denote the i-th frame as $I : \Omega \to \mathbb{R}^+$. It can be observed, for example in Figure 2 in Section 3 below, that the cells appear brighter in the image than their background region. Therefore, we opt to use the region based active contour method (Chan-Vese model)[3] for the cell segmentation due to its ability of both extracting the bright region as well as keeping the boundary relative regular/smooth. Mathematically, the contour is modeled as a simple closed curve in Ω,$C : [0, 1] \to \Omega$ with $C(0) = C(1)$. The extraction of the cell boundary is accomplished by computing the curve C minimizing the energy functional $E(C)$ given as [3]:

$$E(C) := \int_{\text{inside } C} |I(x, y) - \mu_1|^2 \, dxdy + \int_{\text{outside } C} |I(x, y) - \mu_2|^2 \, dxdy + \lambda \int_C ds \quad (1)$$

where μ_1 (μ_2) is the average image intensity inside (outside) the close contour C, respectively. The λ is a positive parameter that controls the smoothness of the resulting contour: large positive λ will result in a smooth cell boundary whereas a small positive λ will capture all the boundary details, at the risk of being influenced by the image noise.

The contour C which gives the minimal $E(C)$ is obtained by solving the variational problem under the level set framework [5]. Specifically, in order to achieve fast processing speed, we used the sparse field level set implementation for the level set evolution [6].

2.2. Ca^{2+} Concentration Estimation

The intra-cellular Ca^{2+} is estimated as the cell image intensity ratio between the 340nm channel and the 380nm channel [2]. Assuming that the cells have been extracted via the preceding segmentation procedure, this can be computed as:

$$a = \int_{\text{inside } C} \frac{I_{340nm}(x, y)}{I_{380nm}(x, y)} dxdy \Big/ \int_{\text{inside } C} 1 dxdy \quad (2)$$

After this, we compute the temporal shape variation and find interesting correlation with the shape of the cell, which are detailed below.

2.3. Shape Metric and Correlation with Ca^{2+} Concentration

In order to compare the shapes of the cell at different time points, we have to formalize the definition of the concept of "shape". We adopt the definition of "shape" which measures the geometric property of the object after certain global similarity transformation is removed [7, 8]. Due to the motion of the cell mounting device, such global transformation should be removed from the shape metric computation. After that, the "distance" between two shapes are defined. Various definition for the shape metric have been proposed [9, 10, 11], in this work, the Wasserstein 2-metric derived from the optimal mass transport is used. Mathematically,

$$d(C_1, C_2) = \min_T (W(R_1, T \circ R_2)) \tag{3}$$

where

$$\hat{R}_i(x,y) = \begin{cases} 1 & \text{if } (x,y) \text{ inside } C_i \\ 0 & \text{otherwise} \end{cases}$$
$$R_i(x,y) = \frac{\hat{R}_i(x,y)}{\int_\Omega \hat{R}_i(x,y)dxdy} \tag{4}$$

and T is the optimal similarity transformation aligning R_1 with R_2. It is computed as:

In the equation, the $W(\cdot,\cdot)$ indicates the Wasserstein distance defined as follows. First, we call a diffeomorphism $\mu : \Omega \to \Omega$ *mass preserving* (MP) if $\forall D \subseteq \Omega$ with $(x,y) = \mu(u,v)$, we have:

$$\int_{\mu^{-1}(D)} R_1(u,v)dudv = \int_D R_2(x,y)dxdy. \tag{5}$$

Via change of variables, this can be rewritten as

$$\det(J_\mu(x,y))R_2(\mu(x,y)) = R_1(x,y), \forall (x,y) \in \Omega \tag{6}$$

where $J_\mu(x,y)$ is the Jacobian of μ at (x,y). This is referred to as the *Jacobian equation*. This equation is highly nonlinear, and may have many solutions. The objective here is to compute the following distance and find the corresponding optimal transportation map (if it exists), defined in terms of the L^p Kantorovich-Wasserstein functional [4]:

$$W(R_1, R_2) = \inf_{\mu \in MP} \left(\int_\Omega |\mu(x,y) - (x,y)|^p R_1(x,y) dx dy \right) \quad (7)$$

The minimization problem defined Equation (7) is highly non-linear and is difficult to solve. The quadratic version of this problem ($p = 2$ in Eq. (7)) has been extensively studied and has a number of approaches devoted to its numerical solution; see [12, 13, 14, 15] and the references therein. Previously, by representing the masses as sum of Dirac delta functions, the linear programming can then be employed in solving the problem [12]. Such scheme is also used to model cell nuclei evolution [15]. However, for 2D images of the size $N \times N$, the complexity of such scheme is $O(N^4)$, which is computationally very heavy for large N. Benamou and Brenier took a different path by casting the original problem to a computational fluid mechanics one [13]. Also in the continuum, Haker et al., [14] took another approach. They first constructed a mass preserving map μ_0 not necessarily minimizing the cost in Equation 7. Then, such initial map was iteratively processed so as to remove its curl component accomplished via a non-local first order partial differential equation. For a given mass-preserving initial mapping, the solution of the equation does indeed asymptotically converge to the optimal map [16], but numerically may have a problem that if the initial mapping is "far" from the final optimal mapping. In such a case, the scheme may require many iteration steps to sufficiently reduce the curl. To address such problems, Haber *et al.* discretized the problem first and then formulated a consistent numerical scheme in the discrete domain using sequential quadratic programming [17].

In the quadratic case, one can show that there exists a unique strictly convex function $\tilde{\Psi} : \Omega \rightarrow \Omega$ such that the optimal mapping $\tilde{\mu}$ is the gradient of $\tilde{\Psi}$, i.e., $\tilde{\mu} = \nabla \tilde{\Psi}$ [18]. Plugging this into Equation 6 we have:

$$\det(H_{\tilde{\Psi}}(x,y)) R_2(\nabla \tilde{\Psi}(x,y)) = R_1(x,y), \quad \forall (x,y) \in \Omega \quad (8)$$

where $H_{\tilde{\Psi}}$ is the Hessian of $\tilde{\Psi}$ and Equation 8 is the Monge-Ampere equation. Following [19], $\tilde{\Psi}$ can be solved iteratively by:

$$\frac{\partial \Psi}{\partial t} = \log \left(\frac{\det(H_{\tilde{\Psi}}(x,y)) R_2(\nabla_{(x,y)} \Psi(x,y))}{R_1(x,y)} \right) \quad (9)$$

When Ψ converges to $\tilde{\Psi}$, we have the optimal mapping $\tilde{\mu} = \nabla_{(x,y)} \Psi$, where $\nabla_{(x,y)}$ is the spatial gradient operator.

2.4. Overall Algorithm

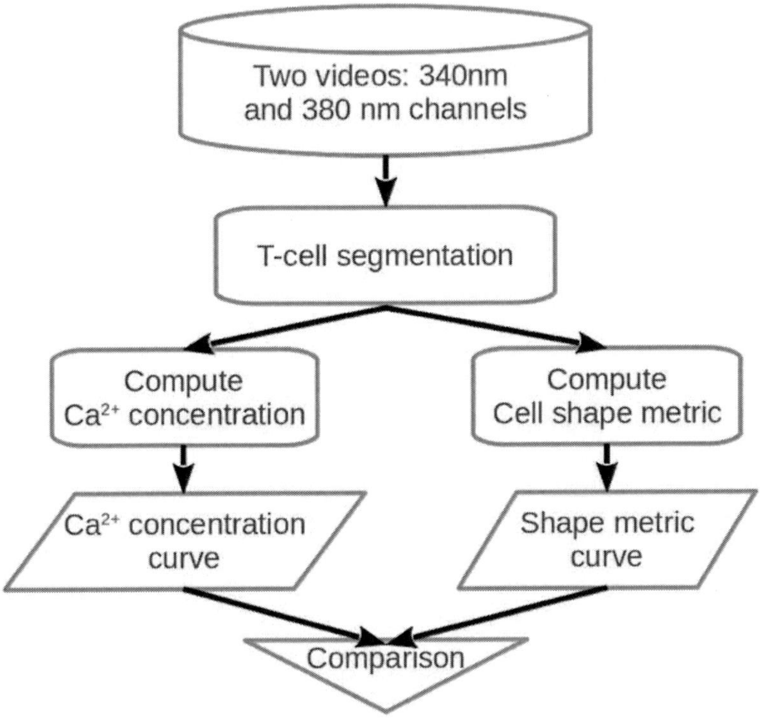

Figure 1. Overall flow chart of the proposed algorithm.

Given a series of images (video), we present the overall algorithm for the entire processing pipeline as shown in Figure 1. Specifically, the input to the processing pipeline consists of two video sequences $I_{340nm}(x, y, t)$ and $I_{380nm}(x, y, t)$ (340 nm and 380 nm channels, respectively). The cell segmentation algorithm in Section 2.1 is used to extract the T-cells in each frame of the two video sequences. Then, the Ca^{2+} concentration in each frame is computed and is denoted by $a(t)$. In parallel, the shape of the T-cell in each subsequent frame is compared with that in the first frame, and is denoted as $S(t) := W(R(t), R(t_0))$. Since we are interested in the trends of $a(t)$ and $S(t)$, not their absolute values, they are normalized by dividing their respective ranges (the difference between maximum and minimum values). Finally, the normalized $a(t)$ and $S(t)$ are compared to show the correlation.

3. Experimental Results

3.1. Cell Extraction

We show in Figure 2 several frames from the video indicating the image condition, cell extraction results, and the shape variance between frames.

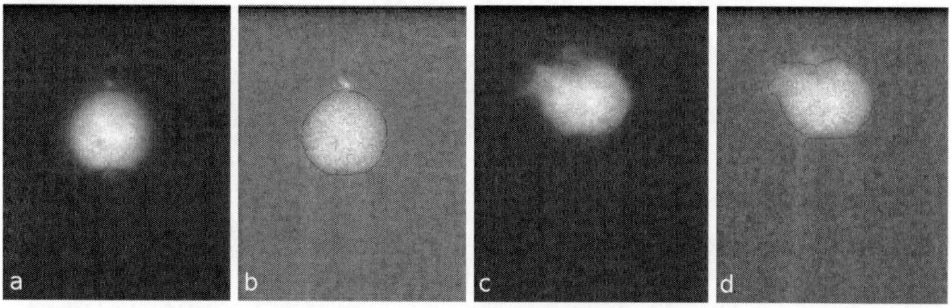

Figure 2. Frame 10 or 380nm (a) and 340nm (b) channels. Frame 115 or 380nm (c) and 340nm (d) channels. The red contours indicate the extracted cell boundaries. Note that the bright spot on top of the cell is glass beads and is correctly excluded from the cell region. The significant shape change between the frames can be observed.

3.2. Shape and Ca^{2+} Correlation

The algorithm is tested on a total of 20 data cases. Among them, three results are picked at random and are shown below. From these figures and similarly on others not shown here because of lack of space, we can observe a positive correlation between the two curves. Moreover, it is interesting to observe that the Ca^{2+} concentration change often precedes the shape change. This is more evident when there is a relatively significant change in both curves, such as in Figure 3 around 270-th frame and Figure 4 around 110-th frame.

4. Conclusion and Discussion

In this work we proposed a complete pipeline for image and shape analysis for the fluorescent T-cell images. In particular, we have used the Wasserstein 2-

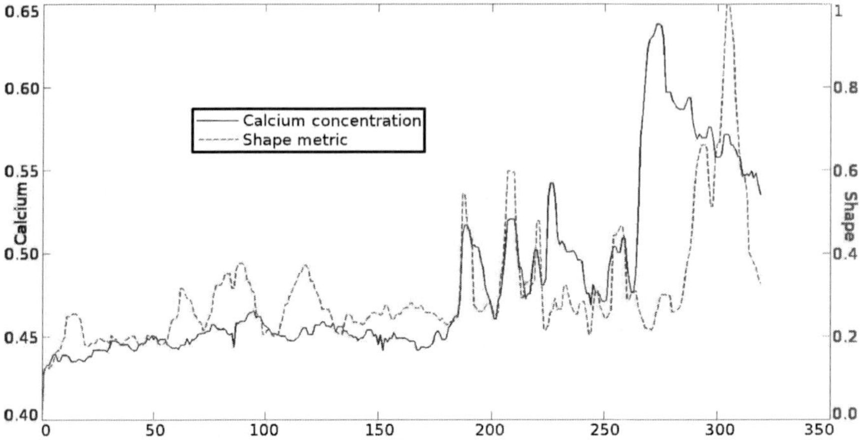

Figure 3. The Ca^{2+} (red) and shape metric (blue) curves and their respective regression lines. Case 1.

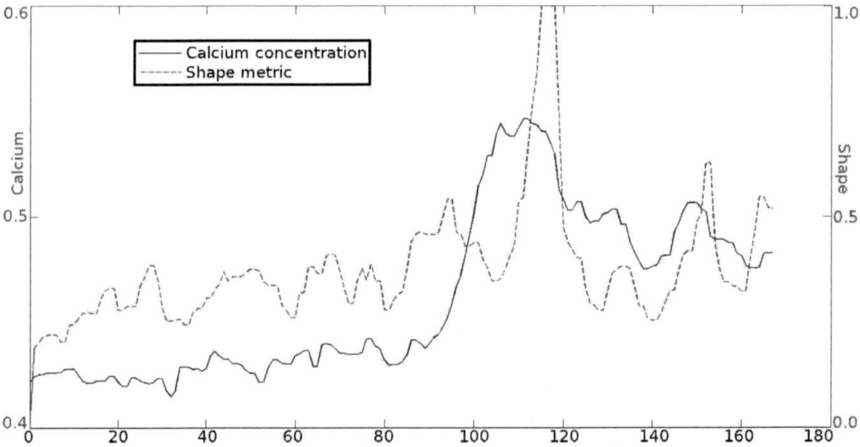

Figure 4. The Ca^{2+} (red) and shape metric (blue) curves and their respective regression lines. Case 2.

metric to measure the shape variation of the T-cells, which shows an interesting correlation with the intracellular calcium concentration.

It is also noted that since both the Ca^{2+} concentration and the shape metric computation depends upon the segmentation of the T-cells, we must consider

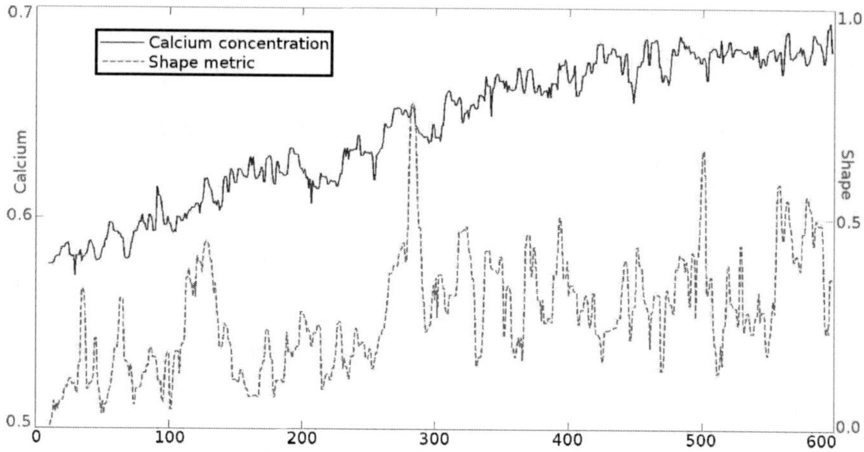

Figure 5. The Ca^{2+} (red) and shape metric (blue) curves and their respective regression lines. Case 3.

the question of whether the correlation between the two measures is caused by the common segmentation upon which they are based. One possible way to verify this is to utilize other methods to compute the Ca^{2+} concentration so that the generation of the two curves are decoupled. In this manner, we plan to further examine the correspondence found in this work. Another future research direction involves the quantitative analysis of the correlation between the Ca^{2+} concentration and the shape metric.

References

[1] Patrick G Hogan, Richard S Lewis, and Anjana Rao. Molecular basis of calcium signaling in lymphocytes: Stim and orai. *Annual review of immunology*, 28:491, 2010.

[2] Grzegorz Grynkiewicz, Martin Poenie, and Roger Y Tsien. A new generation of ca2+ indicators with greatly improved fluorescence properties. *Journal of Biological Chemistry*, 260(6):3440–3450, 1985.

[3] T.F. Chan and L.A. Vese. Active contours without edges. *Image Processing, IEEE Transactions on*, 10(2):266–277, 2001.

[4] Cédric Villani. *Optimal Transport: Old and New*, volume 338. Springer, 2008.

[5] S. Osher and J.A. Sethian. Fronts propagating with curvature-dependent speed: algorithms based on hamilton-jacobi formulations. *Journal of computational physics*, 79(1):12–49, 1988.

[6] Ross T Whitaker. A level-set approach to 3d reconstruction from range data. *International Journal of Computer Vision*, 29(3):203–231, 1998.

[7] C.G. Small. *The statistical theory of shape*. Springer Verlag, 1996.

[8] I.L. Dryden and K.V. Mardia. *Statistical shape analysis*. John Wiley & Sons, 1998.

[9] M.I. Miller. Computational anatomy: shape, growth, and atrophy comparison via diffeomorphisms. *NeuroImage*, 23:S19–S33, 2004.

[10] Y. Gao, T. Riklin-Raviv, and S. Bouix. Shape analysis, a field in need of careful validation. *Human Brain Mapping*, 2014.

[11] Y. Gao and S. Bouix. Signed Poisson map for shape analysis. In *Proceedings of the International Symposium on Biomedical Imaging (ISBI)*, 2014.

[12] T. Kaijser. Computing the Kantorovich distance for images. *Journal of Mathematical Imaging and Vision*, 9(2):173–191, 1998.

[13] J.D. Benamou and Y. Brenier. A computational fluid mechanics solution to the Monge-Kantorovich mass transfer problem. *Numerische Mathematik*, 84(3):375–393, 2000.

[14] S. Haker, L. Zhu, A. Tannenbaum, and S. Angenent. Optimal mass transport for registration and warping. *International Journal of Computer Vision*, 60(3):225–240, 2004.

[15] Wei Wang, John A Ozolek, Dejan Slepcev, Ann B Lee, Cheng Chen, and Gustavo K Rohde. An optimal transportation approach for nuclear structure-based pathology. *IEEE Transactions on Medical Imaging*, 30(3):621–631, 2011.

[16] S. Angenent, Haker S., and Tannenbaum A. Minimizing flows for the monge–kantorovich problem. SIAM J. Math. Analysis, 35:61–97, 2003.

[17] E. Haber, T. Rehman, and A. Tannenbaum. An efficient numerical method for the solution of the l2 optimal mass transfer problem. *SIAM Journal on Imaging Science*, 32(1):197–211, 2010.

[18] Y. Brenier. Polar factorization and monotone rearrangement of vector-valued functions. *Comm. on pure and applied mathematics*, 44(4):375–417, 1991.

[19] M.M. Sulman, JF Williams, and R.D. Russell. An efficient approach for the numerical solution of the monge-ampère equation. *Applied Numerical Mathematics*, 61(3):298–307, 2011.

EDITOR'S CONTACT INFORMATION

Dr. Xiaojun Chen
Institute of Biomedical Manufacturing and Life Quality Engineering
School of Mechanical Engineering,
Shanghai Jiao Tong University,
Shanghai, China
Email: xiaojunchen@163.com

INDEX

D

E

J

K

L

M

N

O

P

Q

R

S

W

X

Z